DISCOVER THE HEALTH SECRET OF THE TROPICS!

Coconuts may make you think of rich desserts—and calories—but the truth is far more slimming! Coconut oil contains a healthy fat that can help boost your weight-loss potential and bring you vibrant health. Simply adding a small amount of this fat-busting oil to your favorite low-carb foods can help you drop those extra pounds. You'll feel better, look better, and be able to maintain your new weight with ease.

With dozens of mouthwatering dishes, no deprivation, and so many health benefits, no diet delivers as much as . . .

THE COCONUT DIET

"An important book . . . exceptional . . . In a clear and engaging style that's an actual pleasure to read, Calbom shows why coconut oil is an incredible health food."

—Dr. Joseph Mercola,
author of the natural-health bestseller
The Total Health Program

THE COCONUT DIET

The SECRET INGREDIENT That Helps You LOSE WEIGHT While You Eat Your Favorite Foods

Cherie Calbom

with John Calbom

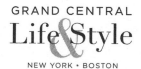

GRAND CENTRAL
Life & Style

NEW YORK • BOSTON

The program herein is not intended to replace the services of trained health professionals, or be a substitute for medical advice. You are advised to consult with your health care professional with regard to matters relating to your health, and in particular regarding matters that may require diagnosis or medical attention.

The Insulin Resistance Quiz at the end of chapter 2, from *Blood Sugar Blues* by Miryam Erlich Williamsen, is printed by arrangement with Walker & Company.

The Fibromyalgia Syndrome Questionnaire at the end of chapter 5 appears courtesy of Kenneth L. Bakken, D.O., fibromyalgia specialist, Bayview Medical Clinic, Tacoma, Washington.

Grand Central Life & Style
Hachette Book Group
237 Park Avenue
New York, NY 10017

www.HachetteBookGroup.com

Printed in the United States of America

Originally published in hardcover by Hachette Book Group.
First Trade Edition: January 2006
10 9 8 7 6 5

Grand Central Life & Style is an imprint of Grand Central Publishing.
The Grand Central Life & Style name and logo are trademarks of Hachette Book Group, Inc.

The publisher is not responsible for websites (or their content) that are not owned by the publisher.

The Library of Congress has cataloged the hardcover edition as follows:
Calbom, Cherie.
     The coconut diet : the secret ingredient that helps you lose weight while you eat your favorite foods / Cherie Calbom with John Calbom.—1st Warner Books ed.
          p. cm.
     Includes bibliographical references.
     ISBN 0-446-57716-2
     1. Reducing diets.   2. Coconut oil—Health aspects.   I. Calbom, John.   II. Title.
     RM222.2.C225 2005
     613.2'5—dc22   2004017361

Book design by Giorgetta Bell McRee

ISBN 978-0-446-69345-5 (pbk.)

Contents

Introduction   vii

PART I The Basis for The Coconut Diet   1

Chapter 1 *Weight Loss Secrets of the Tropics*   3
Chapter 2 *The Carbohydrate Conundrum*   17
Chapter 3 *The Big Fat Misconception*   41
Chapter 4 *Thyroid Health: A Weight Loss Advantage*   59
Chapter 5 *Special Help When Diets Don't Work*   81

PART II The Coconut Diet   111

Chapter 6/Phase I *The 21-Day Weight Loss Kickoff*   113
Chapter 7/Phase II *Cleansing—A Weight Loss Advantage*   213
Chapter 8/Phase III *Introducing Healthy Carbs*   235
Chapter 9/Phase IV *Maintaining Your Healthy Weight*   273

Resources   297

Notes   304

Acknowledgments   311

Index   313

Introduction

You may have tried nearly every diet available. Or maybe this is the first time you've decided to lose weight. No matter what your needs or your successes or failures, you will be pleased to know that this is *the* diet that has worked for many people—*when nothing else would*! You won't be disappointed by The Coconut Diet.

Now, if you're thinking you have to sprinkle coconut flakes on everything you eat, that's not what this diet is about. Though The Coconut Diet does incorporate a number of recipes that include coconut milk or coconut flakes, the diet is mostly about coconut oil. You can eat many of your favorite foods such as fish, chicken, beef, lamb, turkey, and vegetables prepared with coconut oil. You can even enjoy the Low-Carb Coconut Smoothie and still melt away the pounds!

The secret ingredient that has promoted such phenomenal weight loss success for many people is the oil of the coconut. Coconut oil works wonders when combined with a low-carb diet because it is made up of medium-chain triglycerides (MCTs) that burn up quickly in the body—a lot like kindling on a fire; this helps improve metabolism. And, there's plenty of research to back up that statement in the pages that follow.

Thousands have discovered the weight loss miracle of coconut oil added to a low-carbohydrate, lean-protein diet. Many of these people had tried various weight loss diets with little or no success; they became discouraged and disappointed. When they added coconut oil—two to three tablespoons a day—to a healthy, low-carbohydrate diet, to their surprise—the weight came off without effort!

THE DIET THAT WORKS!

With the exciting 21-day low-carb, coconut diet meal plan and dozens of scrumptious recipes, you are on your way to a *new you*. You can enjoy your favorite low-carb foods prepared with coconut oil. You'll be amazed at how delicious your food tastes. That's all you have to do. Just think, you can eat great-tasting food *and* lose weight!

Does this sound too good to be true? You'll hear from scores of people who have tried The Coconut Diet and lost. They not only lost weight, they lost a host of health problems to boot!

The Coconut Diet is fun, easy, delicious, and exciting. It's exciting because it produces results without struggle or deprivation. Without cravings or climbing the kitchen wall. You'll feel satisfied after eating, you'll enjoy your food, and you'll be smiling when you step on the scale.

The Coconut Diet is one of the best-kept secrets of the tropics and now it's yours.

You may be thinking, "Yikes! Coconut oil! Isn't that a saturated fat—something that's unhealthy?" Let me reassure you that people eating traditional diets rich in coconut oil have lived for centuries free of many modern diseases including obesity and heart disease that plague Western cultures. Coconut oil, and saturated fat in general, have gotten a bad rap. It all started with faulty studies decades ago. You can read more about that in chapter 3.

Right now, get ready to enjoy great-tasting food made with the best weight loss ingredient ever—coconut oil.

WHAT IS THE COCONUT DIET?

The Coconut Diet encourages the consumption of healthy fats—especially coconut oil, which has unique properties—that increase the body's metabolism, leading to weight loss. The Coconut Diet is predominantly low in the carbohydrates that pack on weight, such as refined grains, potatoes, sugars, desserts, and alcohol. It is high in antioxidant-rich vegetables that help prevent disease. It doesn't toss the carrots out with the potato chips because all carbohydrates are not created equal! You'll learn which carbs are healthy and which are not.

The Coconut Diet teaches you how to eat healthy for a lifetime by including good carbohydrates, lean proteins, and healthy fats with the secret ingredient: two to three tablespoons of coconut oil each day.

You'll lose weight. You'll lose cravings. And you'll get healthy— maybe healthier than you've been in years.

Phase I: The 21-Day Weight Loss Kickoff

Phase I, which is the fast track, is the strictest portion of the program, but the results are worth it. During these 21 days you should lose 10 or more pounds without much effort.

There's no starvation. No deprivation. These are the basics:

You will consume two to three tablespoons of virgin coconut oil each and every day. The only other oil I recommend is extra virgin olive oil.

You'll eat lean protein—fish, chicken, turkey, lamb, beef, eggs, nuts, and cheese.

You'll eat plenty of vegetables, especially the brightly colored veggies that are highest in antioxidants.

You'll drink 8 to 10 eight-ounce glasses of water each day and herbal tea. You'll learn why it's best to avoid coffee as much as possible.

Now does that sound difficult? Of course not!

There's even a 1-Day Vegetable Juice Cleanse for those who want to accelerate their weight loss by incorporating a day of vegetable juicing. This is an optional day. You can include this day for one, two, or all three weeks. Not only will you speed up your weight loss, you'll feel incredibly energized and cleansed.

With The Coconut Diet, you should start looking younger and trimmer—and feeling better—in no time at all.

Phase II: Cleansing

The Coconut Diet may be the only low-carb diet that offers four weeks of cleansing for weight loss and revitalization. This part of the weight loss program is not mandatory, but if you are interested in reshaping and rejuvenating your body, the cleansing programs will produce results that nothing else ever could—like getting rid of a protruding tummy or cellulite (that lumpy, bumpy, orange peel–looking skin).

Before you decide to skip over the cleansing programs, I suggest you read a little about what each program can do for you and how it can affect your weight loss. Then, you just might decide to try a few weeks of cleansing. I think you'll be happily surprised with how you feel and with your weight loss success.

Phase III: Introducing Healthy Carbs

Phase III slowly adds back healthy carbs. With a one-week menu plan and recipes that include whole grains, potatoes, squash, fruit, and healthy desserts, you will have more variety, but you'll eat these foods sparingly until you reach your weight loss goal.

Typically, in this phase, you'll lose one to two pounds per week. When you reach your goal weight, you'll be able to add a few more of these foods each week.

If you really splurge for holidays, vacations, or special occasions, I'll show you a trick to quickly lose weight and cleanse away the junk—the 1-Day Vegetable Juice Cleanse.

Phase IV: Maintaining Your Healthy Weight

Phase IV signals the achievement of your weight loss goals. Now you can eat more healthy carbohydrates, and by this time, you'll be in the habit of choosing the right ones. To continue your program, a one-week menu plan with recipes introduces a full complement of healthy carbs. If you eat too many of them occasionally and put on a few pounds, you can go back to Phase I, II, or III until you've lost the extra weight. If you binge on junk food during a stressful time, you can schedule a vegetable juice–cleanse day. This is the plan you can maintain for the rest of your life.

A NEW EATING STYLE FOR A HEALTHIER LIFE

When you complete this program, you should have changed your internal chemistry and established new food-choice habits. The cravings and urges that once lured you to the refrigerator for foods you didn't even want should be gone. And that could be forever—if you make this style of eating a way of life.

Best of all—you will become healthier. Just like many of the folks whose stories you'll read in this book, you too may feel better on this program than you've ever felt. You'll have more energy to enjoy each and every day. And, you'll stand the greatest chance of preventing such serious diseases as cancer, diabetes, and heart disease.

You'll want to maintain this diet because feeling healthy, happy, and energetic is something you'll never want to lose, no matter how alluring some foods might be. Let's face it, feeling and looking fabulous are what most people strive for every day they're alive.

PART I

The Basis for
The Coconut Diet

Chapter 1

Weight Loss Secrets of the Tropics

Healthy, trim, energetic, and alive! That's what you can be when you make The Coconut Diet your weight loss secret. With coconut oil, you can watch the pounds melt away. This secret ingredient has promoted great weight loss success for many, many people. You'll learn what makes coconut oil a fast-burning fat and how that increases metabolism and promotes weight loss. You'll hear from scores of people who have lost weight—for many, lots of weight—and health problems, too. Most important, you'll experience a diet that works.

Coconut oil received very bad press several decades ago. You'll learn why that was completely unfounded. But first I'd like to tell you how people have eaten in tropical, coconut-growing countries for centuries. You may be surprised to learn that a high-saturated-fat diet is the reason why most tropical islanders remain trim and healthy all their lives when they stick to eating their traditional foods rich in coconut oil.

COCONUT: A DIETARY STAPLE IN THE TROPICS

In tropical cultures where coconut is often a staple in the diet and traditional foods the local fare, one can find a preponderance of healthy, trim people, even though their diet is high in calories and fat—particularly saturated fat from coconut oil.

Prior to World War II (and for several decades afterward), people who ate traditional foods in countries such as the Philippines were rarely sick or overweight. The diet in most communities consisted mainly of rice, coconuts, vegetables, root crops (especially garlic and ginger), herbs, and meat that was raised locally. Many people ground their own rice by hand, leaving intact most of the bran and nutrients.

Food processing changed following World War II. Rice mills replaced the need to hand-mill rice. These first mills were "crude" and did not polish the rice; thus people still ate healthy high-fiber grains. Later, the mills became more sophisticated and polished the rice, making it bright white, stripped of the bran and most of the nutrients.

The food consumed prior to World War II would be considered "organic" by today's standards. People had no access to chemical fertilizers or pesticides. The animals, such as chickens, cows, and goats, all grazed on natural green vegetation.

Coconut and coconut oil were used daily. The usual diet was quite high in fat—the saturated fat from the coconut. Many people made their coconut oil by hand using either the traditional boiling or fermentation method. For many Filipinos and other inhabitants of the tropics, the traditional method of making coconut oil fell out of vogue after World War II. Coconut plants and coconut oil mills were established for the booming baking industry in the United States. Refined coconut oil made its way into the local economy. Though some still made coconut oil the "old-fashioned" way, many people chose to buy the cheaper, odorless, refined coconut oil, which was readily available in the marketplace. But even the refined coconut oil made from copra (dried coconut meat) was done through a mechanical pressing that did not use solvents (chemicals).

Pharmaceuticals were introduced in the Philippines and other tropical countries after World War II, but people in many rural communities could not afford them. They had their own traditions of dealing with sicknesses using local herbs and coconut oil. When people did visit the doctor, which was rare, it was usually not for the ailments that plague Westerners today such as diabetes, cancer, heart disease, and thyroid problems. These illnesses were virtually un-

Since entering menopause, my body really changed and I developed fat on my belly, the underside of my arms, my chin—all kinds of places that I never had fat before. I dieted and dieted. I always ate low-fat and low-calorie foods and never really lost any weight until I tried low-carb dieting with coconut oil. There are many low-carb diets but this is the only one that has worked for me. I eat all the fat [virgin coconut oil] I want and I don't worry about it. I now have only 10 pounds to go to be where I was in college. The virgin coconut oil has also been very good for my skin. I know that exercise and virgin coconut oil will help me get rid of the last 10 pounds.

—*Laurel*

known prior to the 1980s, when Western foods began to saturate the market. People visited the doctor to treat wounds or because of sicknesses common in the tropics, such as malaria, dengue (tropical diseases transmitted by mosquitoes), and diarrhea.

This picture of life in rural tropical communities is typical for those who grew up in the 1950s, '60s, and '70s (and before) eating traditional foods with an abundance of saturated fat from coconut oil. Sadly, this way of life is no longer the norm. Beginning in the mid-1970s, demand for coconut oil dropped so low that most coconut farmers could no longer afford to support their families on the income of coconut harvests. Many people left their farms and moved to the cities to find better employment, where they adopted Western-style diets.

Cheaper, mass-produced foods have replaced most of the local traditional fare people used to raise themselves. Snack foods and other fast foods made with hydrogenated coconut oil, which keeps them solid at sweltering tropical temperatures, made their way onto store shelves. Polished rice grown with chemical fertilizers is now a staple. Soft drinks loaded with refined sugars and chemicals are found on nearly every street corner. These drinks have replaced the natural buko juice—water from the inside of the coconuts—that earlier generations enjoyed. Even the coconut water drinks, once natural and healthy, are now loaded with refined sugar. The traditional high-fat, low-refined-carbohydrate diet has been replaced with many refined, high-carb substitutes.

In the 1950s it was very rare to see anyone in the tropics who was considered overweight, and almost never did people see someone who was considered obese. Since traditional diets have changed in these countries and coconut oil has been exchanged for refined oils, weight problems and diseases are on the rise.

Researchers have discovered that cultures that make coconut oil part of their daily diet enjoy great health. Research on the benefits of coconut oil also suggests that by making this oil part of your daily diet, you can also experience the weight management and health benefits long enjoyed by people of the tropics. In the pages that follow you will find a preponderance of research and supporting evidence as to why coconut oil is such a weight loss wonder.

THE WEIGHT LOSS SECRET

The weight loss *secret* is in the chain—the chain of molecules that make up the fat of coconut oil. These shorter-chain fatty acids that dominate coconut oil are known as medium-chain triglycerides (MCTs). They burn up quickly in the body. They're a lot like adding kindling to a fire, rather than a big damp log. That's the secret to coconut oil's weight loss success!

Following rapid breakdown and absorption in the intestinal tract, MCTs are transported directly to the liver. Once there, they freely enter the mitochondria (the energy-producing elements of the cell) and are rapidly converted to ketones, which are almost immediately converted into energy.[1] On the other hand, long-chain triglycerides (LCTs), which comprise most other oils, are transported from the intestines as chylomicrons (relatively large fat droplets). They are eventually dumped into the bloodstream near the heart.[2] These fat droplets must then be transported through the entire body before they reach the liver.

This difference in metabolism means that the body treats MCTs in a completely different manner than the way it deals with other fats. LCTs are slow to metabolize in the body, and as a result, are more easily stored as fat. MCTs, on the other hand, rapidly burn for energy use, thus are less likely to contribute to fat storage.[3] If you consider your body's metabolism to be like an oil furnace, eating LCTs is like adding oil to the storage tank, whereas consuming MCTs is like pumping fuel from the delivery truck right into the furnace. Less is stored; more is burned.

Because the LCT molecule is so large, the body cannot process it very efficiently; it prefers to simply store it in adipose tissue (fat cells). On the other hand, MCTs can be rapidly converted into energy. Here's how it works: The body removes the carbon atoms two at a time and transforms them into ketones, which are high-energy molecules that pass easily back into the bloodstream and are carried quickly to the cells. Once in the cells, they can be rapidly turned into ATP (adenosine triphosphate), the energy molecules of the body. Eating MCTs could be likened to putting premium fuel in the gas tank of your car—it burns more efficiently.

Thermogenesis is the rate at which the body burns fuel for energy. A unique quality of MCTs is their ability to increase the rate at which the body burns fat for fuel. This could account for the trim, healthy constitution of most Pacific Islanders who eat a diet high in traditional fats that are primarily composed of MCTs.[4]

One of the most popular epidemiological (population) studies was conducted in the South Pacific islands of Pukapuka and Tokelau near New Zealand. The studies began in the 1960s before either island was exposed to Western refined foods. These populations ate only natural foods, and coconut foods were the most prevalent, being consumed at each meal in one form or another.

While most people in Western countries were getting 30 to 40 percent of their calories from fat, these islanders averaged between 50 and 60 percent of their calories from fat, most of that being saturated fat from coconuts. The overall health of both groups of

I have been using coconut oil for about six weeks and following a healthy diet with plenty of organic fruits, vegetables, and meat, and few manufactured foods. I eat only a small amount of carbs—some pasta or rice, but only one time a week, if that. No bread, only Ry-Krisp. The only fats I use are olive oil and coconut oil. I have lost three inches off my hips and two inches off my upper arms so far. Hurrah! I am delighted; [it's been] so easy eating great food. Everybody can see an increase in my energy and mobility level[s], which have been low since I was injured in a car accident some years ago. I don't know the actual pounds [lost], but I'm not really hung up on that. A tape measure and my clothes [let me know how I'm doing]. I'm feeling *great*!

—*Liz*

islanders was extremely good compared with Western standards. There were no signs of kidney disease or hypothyroidism that might influence fat levels. There was no hypercholesterolemia (high blood cholesterol) either. All inhabitants were lean and healthy despite a very high saturated-fat diet. In fact, the populations as a whole had ideal weight-to-height ratios as compared to the body mass index (BMI) figures used by doctors and nutritionists. Digestive problems were rare. Constipation was uncommon; they averaged two or more bowel movements a day. Atherosclerosis, heart disease, colitis, colon cancer, hemorrhoids, ulcers, diverticulosis, and appendicitis are conditions with which they were unfamiliar.[5]

HEALTH SECRETS OF THE TROPICS

Not only do MCTs raise the body's metabolism leading to weight loss, they promote health as well. The health secret of the tropics is the same as the weight loss secret—the fatty acids of coconut oil lead to healing and disease prevention. The incredible health properties of MCTs were researched and documented by Dr. Jon Kabara as far back as 1966.

The most predominant MCT in coconut oil is lauric acid. The lipid researcher Dr. Jon Kabara says, "Never before in the history of man is it so important to emphasize the value of lauric oils. These medium-chain fats in coconut oil are similar to fats in mother's milk and have similar nutriceutical [medical food] effects. It is the fat content that offers the health benefits. The medium-chain fatty acids and monoglycerides found primarily in coconut oil and mother's milk have miraculous healing power."[6] Outside of human breast milk, coconut oil is nature's most abundant source of lauric acid and other medium-chain fatty acids. MCTs have been part of infant formulas and hospital formulas for many years.

Much of the research completed on coconut oil, and, specifically, lauric acid, has centered around the antimicrobial and antiviral properties of this unique fatty acid. Today, many strains of bacteria are becoming resistant to antibiotics. Studies have shown that antibiotics are generally ineffective in treating viral infections. When

---

I'm a nurse working at a natural alternatives wellness center in Missouri. I use virgin coconut oil as a foundational product for all of my clients. It is one of the most powerful supplements I have ever worked with. I have been in the healing arts for 30 years and natural approaches for 20 years. Most of my clients are able to use three to four tablespoons [of coconut oil] per day from the start with amazing results such as improved immune system and energy level, stabilized blood sugar, improved thyroid function, weight loss, increased mental clarity, and improved emotional/mental stability. In addition to being a wonderful supplement, coconut oil is a basic food, which should replace all other oils in the diet. I don't know of any other product that covers so many bases—and it tastes great too!

—*Marie*

lauric acid is consumed in the diet, either in human breast milk or in coconut oil, it forms a monoglyceride called "monolaurin," which has been shown to help destroy a variety of lipid-coated viruses, including HIV, herpes simplex virus-1, vesicular stomatitis virus, influenza, and cytomegalovirus[7] and a variety of bacteria such as helicobacter pylori. Additionally, there is evidence that the MCTs in coconut oil kill yeast infections such as *Candida albicans.*[8]

TRADITIONAL TROPICAL DIETS

A number of studies on the effects of diets heavy in saturated fat offer evidence that coconut oil helps maintain optimal health and weight levels. For example, Dr. Weston Price, a dentist who conducted a number of studies in the 1930s among Pacific Islanders, spent significant time examining the islanders' traditional diets. He looked at their general health, and specifically their dental health, as compared with islanders who ate more modern diets consisting of refined foods.[9]

Doctor Price found that those islanders who ate a traditional diet consisting of high concentrations of coconut were in very good health and were not obese, even though they had a very high-fat diet. Those who traded commercially with Western countries and ate more refined foods high in carbohydrates suffered from common Western diseases, including dental decay.

A study conducted in India by the Department of Medicine, at Safdarjang Hospital in New Delhi, compared traditional cooking oils and fats, like coconut oil and ghee (clarified butter), which are rich in saturated fats, with modern oils like sunflower or safflower, which are mostly polyunsaturated, in relation to the prevalence of heart disease and type 2 diabetes. They found that heart disease and diabetes had actually *increased* after a *decrease* in the consumption of the traditional oils like coconut oil and ghee. It is generally accepted that weight gain is typically associated with heart disease and diabetes. They concluded that these newer "heart-friendly" oils like sunflower and safflower possess an undesirable ratio of omega-6 fatty acids to omega-3 fatty acids. Other similar studies in the region indicate that the sole use or excessive intake of these modern vegetable oils can be detrimental to one's health.[10]

P. K. Thampan, the former chief coconut development officer of the Coconut Development Board in India, made similar discoveries in his study of traditional cultures that consumed large amounts of coconut. In his book *Facts and Fallacies About Coconut Oil,* Thampan shows that coconut oil consumption is unrelated to coronary heart disease mortality and morbidity, which is contrary to what is taught in many countries. Observations recorded in countries where palm kernel and coconut oil form major dietary components have shown a longer life expectancy at birth than in countries with a negligible intake of tropical oils. There are also instances of longer life expectancy in predominantly coconut-consuming areas within the same country where less coconut is consumed.[11]

Dr. P. Rethinam and Muhartoyo wrote in the *Jakarta Post* (2003) that before 1950, heart attacks were uncommon in Sri Lanka. However, hospital admission rates for heart attacks grew dramatically

I read a coconut oil article in *Woman's World* magazine [May 2003] and decided to give [coconut oil] a try. I have suffered horrible pain and fatigue from fibromyalgia for about 10 years. Pain pills weren't much help and they added to the fogged-brain feeling. Within five days of starting the coconut oil—four tablespoons per day, sometimes more—I was almost completely pain free. [Prior to that] I could not drive more than an hour without being in tears. We just got back from a nine-state, nine-day driving vacation and I drove pain free the entire way. I was never diagnosed with thyroid problems, but had many of the symptoms, and that is much better, too. I lost 17 pounds within the first 10 days on the oil. I cannot say enough about it. I am 60 years old and certainly never expected to get the super results I have received.

—*Joyce*

from 1970 to 1992, which might be explained in part by the fact that coconut consumption has gone down from an average of 132 nuts per person per year in 1952 to 90 per person per year in 1991.[12]

HOW DID COCONUT OIL GET SUCH A BAD REPUTATION?

If coconut oil doesn't cause heart problems, but, in fact, promotes wellness, where did the notion come from that this oil is so very detrimental to our health? The answer involves a brief history lesson.

During World War II, when the Japanese occupied most of the Philippines and the South Pacific, supplies of coconut oil were cut off for several years. Americans were forced to turn to alternative sources of cooking oils, and this is when many of the polyunsaturated oils began to make their way to the marketplace.

Beginning in the 1950s, public opinion toward saturated fats in general, and then later toward coconut oil in particular, began to turn negative. The anti–saturated fat theory began in the 1950s, with the steep rise in heart disease. While heart disease probably caused no more than 10 percent of all deaths in the United States prior to the 1920s, by the 1950s it had risen to more than 30 percent. Researchers were looking for the cause of this new threat to health.[13]

Some researchers suggested that cholesterol levels were the problem, and that saturated fats raised cholesterol levels. One study examined the artery plaques found in American soldiers who had died in Korea. With high levels of cholesterol found in artery plaques, some researchers started looking at cholesterol levels found in various foods as a possible cause. Cholesterol is found only in animal foods such as meat, shellfish, cheese, eggs, and butter. Soon a "lipid hypothesis" formed that stated "saturated fat and cholesterol from animal sources raise cholesterol levels in the blood, leading to deposition of cholesterol and fatty material as pathogenic plaques in the arteries." The traditional foods such as butter, eggs, and fat from meats were "out," and the new vegetable oils were seen as heart-healthy replacements.

Research now shows that cholesterol levels in food have only a minor impact or no effect on blood cholesterol levels. Many researchers have rejected the *lipid theory* as a cause of heart disease. The cause of the rapid rise of heart disease in the United States is now attributed to many other factors. See chapter 3, page 56.

After World War II there were significant changes in the American diet, including the kinds of fats Americans began eating. Mary Enig offers insight:

> Butter consumption was declining while the use of vegetable oils, especially oils that had been hardened to resemble butter by a process called hydrogenation, was increasing—dramatically increasing. By 1950 butter consumption had dropped from eighteen pounds per person per year to just over ten. Margarine filled in the gap, rising from about two pounds per person at the turn of the century to about eight. Consumption of vegetable shortening—used in crackers and baked goods— remained relatively steady at about twelve pounds per person per year but vegetable oil consumption had more than tripled— from just under three pounds per person per year to more than ten.[14]

COCONUT OIL BECOMES THE CENTER OF ATTACK

The saturated fats and cholesterol scare soon began to influence mainstream thinking, and before long certain groups started taking aim at the saturated fats found in coconut oil. At one time coconut oil was a significant part of the American diet. Suddenly, consumers were told to avoid *anything* with tropical oils—from theater popcorn to packaged snack foods.

In 1986, the American Soybean Association (ASA) sent out a "Fat Fighter Kit" to soybean farmers that encouraged them to write to government officials and food companies protesting the import of the highly saturated tropical fats of palm and coconut oils.[15] And in 1988, the Center for Science in the Public Interest (CSPI) published a booklet called the "Saturated Fat Attack." Section III, "Those Troublesome Tropical Oils," which encouraged manufacturers to put warnings on food labels against saturated fats. "There were lots of substantive mistakes in the booklet, including errors in the description of the biochemistry of fats and oils and completely erroneous statements about the fat and oil composition of many of the products," writes Dr. Enig.[16]

In 1988, Nebraska millionaire Phil Sokolof joined in the attack by taking out a full-page newspaper ad warning about the dangers of coconut oil. Sokolof was a recovered heart attack patient and the founder of the National Heart Savers Association. His newspaper advertising accused food companies of "poisoning America" by using tropical oils high in saturated fats. He ran a national ad campaign that attacked tropical oils as a health danger by showing a picture of a coconut "bomb" with a lighted wick and cautioning consumers that their health was threatened by coconut oil.[17]

The tropical oil industry, centered in countries like the Philippines, Malaysia, and Indonesia, did not have the financial resources to counter such negative media campaigns. However, many researchers who knew the truth about coconut oil tried to set the record straight, but public opinion was already stacked against saturated fats and tropical oils.

In June of 1988 researchers familiar with tropical oils were called upon to testify before a congressional hearing on tropical oils. "Coconut oil has a neutral effect on blood cholesterol, even in situations where coconut oil is the sole source of fat," reported Dr. George Blackburn, a Harvard Medical School researcher who attended this congressional hearing.

Doctor Enig stated: "These [tropical] oils have been consumed as a substantial part of the diet of many groups for thousands of years with absolutely no evidence of any harmful effects to the populations consuming them."

> I have lost 56 pounds so far and have another 20 to 50 pounds to go. I know I'll get there. I have added coconut oil to a low-carb diet that I've been on for 11 months. I am now off all prescription medications for high blood pressure, asthma, and allergies. My cholesterol levels have improved greatly—triglycerides were 940, and in three months have gone down to 247. I have energy again and can exercise. A year ago I could not walk around the mall without stopping to rest. Now I go day hiking with my hubby. The coconut oil fits perfectly with this way of eating. I have my life back!
>
> —*Dabs*

Dr. C. Everett Koop, the former surgeon general, even called the tropical oil scare "Foolishness!" and added, "but to get the word to commercial interests terrorizing the public about nothing is another matter."[18]

But despite their efforts, the voices of coconut oil defenders were drowned by mainstream media sources informed by members of the edible oil industry and members of the scientific and medical community, thus virtually banishing coconut oil to the margins of the American diet. But this is all about to change with the introduction of The Coconut Diet.

THE TRUTH CAN MAKE YOU TRIM

What we know today, but was not understood in the 1950s, is that hydrogenated and partially hydrogenated vegetable oils contain trans-fatty acids that have been linked to heart disease as well as other health problems. And vegetable oils, which are made up predominantly of LCTs, can cause us to gain weight.

Amid all the hype and hoopla about coconut oil—you now know the full story. Coconut oil is one of the reasons Asians and people of the tropics who eat a traditional diet that includes coconut are typically not overweight and don't usually suffer from diseases that plague Westerners. The secret of the tropics—the key to weight loss and vibrant health—is in eating the right kinds of fats, avoiding refined carbohydrates, and consuming a diet of whole foods.

The 21-day program found in *The Coconut Diet* will help you to make dietary changes for the better and reap the benefits of improved health and weight management. You will lose weight on The Coconut Diet, and the program, meal plans, and recipes will help you put this diet into action.

Chapter 2

The Carbohydrate Conundrum

When I mention the word "carbohydrate," what comes to your mind? If you're like most people, probably sugar and starch. The topic of carbohydrates is certainly confusing for a lot of folks. Do human beings need these sugars and starches or don't they? For decades consumers have been told to eat lots of carbs, making them the highest percentage of their diet, and to limit protein and fat as much as possible. Now, they're being told the opposite.

Because of all the encouragement over the years to eat carbs, Americans have become the primary refined carbohydrate consumers of the world. From bagels, muffins, boxed sugary cereals, and orange juice for breakfast, sweet rolls and doughnuts for coffee break, sandwiches and French fries for lunch, and pasta and bread for dinner, many people have centered their entire day around refined carbs.

Unfortunately, most of the carbs Americans eat are not the healthy, fiber-rich carbohydrates eaten in many other parts of the world; these are simple, refined carbs that have had the fiber and nutrients stripped away. Once ingested, these foods rapidly turn to sugar in the body. And all this sugar, scientists say, make individuals fat and unhealthy.

WHAT ARE CARBOHYDRATES?

Carbohydrates are macronutrients known as sugars, starches, and fiber. A carbohydrate is composed of carbon, hydrogen, and oxygen, and carbohydrates come arranged in three sizes—monosaccharides, disaccharides, and polysaccharides. The monosaccharides and disaccharides are simple carbohydrates such as white sugar. The polysaccharides are complex carbohydrates that include starches, glycogen (a polysaccharide, stored in the liver and easily converted to glucose), and most fiber.

To help you succeed on The Coconut Diet, you'll need an understanding of the difference between the good carbs and the bad.

Simple Carbohydrates: The Bad Ones

When it comes to blood sugar and weight management, simple carbs such as sugar, starch, and refined flour products are the biggest obstacles. These foods have little or no fiber and plenty of readily available sugar. French fries, sweet rolls, pretzels, potato chips, soda pop, milk shakes, ice cream, doughnuts, bagels, alcohol, and most packaged breakfast cereals are all examples of foods that provide high amounts of simple carbs, very few, if any, nutrients, and little to no fiber. They convert to sugar quickly in the bloodstream, which often goes straight to the fat cells.

Some of the simple-carbohydrate foods can catch us off guard—they don't taste sweet, and we may think we're actually eating something healthful. Take a savory-flavored rice cake, for example. It has no fat and not a lot of calories, but look out when it comes to simple carbs—about 12 carbs in each flavored rice cake; plain has about 8 grams of carbs. Many people have felt good about eating three or four of these snack crackers in place of something that has fat in it. But rice cakes are not a good carb choice. They are made of puffed rice, which is high on the glycemic index (an index that shows the rate at which carbohydrates break down to glucose in the bloodstream and turn to sugar). White bread is another example; it doesn't taste sweet either. We may think it's okay when it's French or sourdough bread or a sesame bread stick—at least these forms of white flour have a more sophisticated image than a slice of plain white bread. There's not much difference, however, between eating these breads and a sweet in terms of how quickly they turn to sugar when they are digested.

Your body's primary way of getting rid of sugar is to burn it. What your body can't burn it stores as glycogen. When your glycogen stores are filled up, your body begins storing fat.

"Sugar is a turbo charger—a very hot-burning fuel," says Dr. Ron Rosedale. When you eat a lot of carbohydrates, and particularly simple carbs, your body will convert it quickly to sugar and burn it, and it will stop burning fat.[1] (This is the reason low-carb diets are so effective—they promote fat burning.)

With an emphasis on lots of carb servings every day, our bodies may not get around to fat burning at all. For instance, start the morning with a bowl of cornflakes, one-half cup skim milk, a small banana, and a glass of orange juice. How about a bran muffin for coffee break—that's healthy right? Maybe you choose a sandwich with no mayo for lunch. How about pasta primavera and garlic bread for dinner? And you could end the day with a bowl of plain popcorn for an evening snack.

This looks like a healthy-choice, low-fat-kind-of-day to many people across the United States, but when we add up the carbs, it comes to over 200 grams and most of those are simple carbs. Guidelines for carbs on many low-carb weight loss programs are usually around 30 grams per day. A bran muffin alone has about 28 carb grams.

Is it any wonder that many Americans can't lose weight, have blood sugar problems, and experience insulin resistance? They fill their entire day with one high-carb meal after another, and their blood sugar is bouncing around like a yo-yo.

As you maintain satisfactory blood glucose and insulin levels, the body will not easily store excess carbohydrates as fat, and it will burn existing fat stores faster. As you follow a healthful, low-carb food plan such as The Coconut Diet, you can achieve permanent fat loss and build more muscle.

I have been taking a tablespoon of coconut oil three times daily with meals. Taking the oil with my meals seems to give me a "full feeling" a lot faster. My sweet tooth has practically vanished—and this is from someone who should have bought stock in Hershey's long ago! Ironically, facilitating weight loss was my main reason for trying the coconut oil diet, but with all the wonderful benefits I am experiencing, the weight loss aspect almost seems like an afterthought.

About three days into the routine, I had an energy rush on a Saturday morning that kept me going until well after lunch. I can't believe how much I got done that day! My mental state of mind seemed to be much sharper. I was able to focus on the tasks at hand without getting sidetracked. I was not exhausted at the end of running my errands, which included traipsing around a huge mall. It seemed like I was practically running, rather than the leisurely walking that was formerly my habit. In addition to my energy level, my mood has been very stable—no up and down mood swings—even with the onset of PMS!

My husband commented yesterday on how soft and silky my skin felt, and I have not used any lotion since I started taking the oil. This program also seems to have given my libido a jump start, too.

—*Theresa*

Complex Carbohydrates: The Good Ones

The complex carbohydrates (polysaccharides) are condensed into molecules of starch, glycogen, and cellulose. Starch molecules are rather large; a single starch molecule may contain 3,000 or more glucose units linked together. Starch is the stored form of glucose in a plant. Potatoes, rice and other grains, corn, and legumes are examples of starch. Glycogen is more complex than starch and is found in animal meats, to a limited extent. Cellulose is found primarily in plants and has long, branching chains that are not digestible by human enzymes. Cellulose is also known as insoluble fiber and it is very important in human nutrition, especially for colon health.

Most plant foods have fiber and an abundance of nutrients, particularly the brightly colored vegetables, fruits, sprouts, legumes, herbs, and sea vegetables. These are powerhouses of vitamins, minerals, enzymes, phytochemicals, and fiber. Even on a carb-restricted diet, you can eat large amounts of most vegetables, salad greens, and sprouts and never feel deprived, while maintaining a low-carb intake. The high-fiber content of these foods slows down the rate that sugars enter the bloodstream, thereby lowering insulin secretion. These vegetables, sprouts, herbs, and salad greens will be your primary source of carbohydrates during the first three weeks of The Coconut Diet.

A few vegetables such as potatoes, squash, and parsnips, and fruits such as watermelon, pineapple, and bananas are not good carb choices because they are higher on the glycemic index; they should be avoided in Phases I and II (see chapters 6 and 7).

SWEETENERS: THE GOOD, THE BAD, AND THE DANGEROUS

Sweeteners, no matter what we call them, are still sugars. Only a few sugars are actually good for us, such as fructooligosaccharides and other essential saccharides. But these sugars are rarely, if ever, found in snacks and treats; they are mostly used for medicinal purposes.

Most natural sweeteners such as honey and pure maple sugar are a little better than refined sugars, because they have some nutrients and they aren't bleached and refined; however, they are not healthful in the quantities consumed by the average American. And some sweeteners, namely artificial, can even be dangerous.

> I consider *Candida albicans* a blessing, actually, because it was
> the only thing that motivated me to go off sugar and [on to] a
> low-carb diet. In the process, I lost 100 pounds!
>
> —*Marie*

Sugar can have many detrimental effects on the body. One is suppression of the immune system. Here's how it works: vitamin C has a similar structure to glucose and thus they compete with each other. In the 1970s, scientists found that vitamin C was needed for white blood cells to phagocytize (engulf and digest) bacteria, cancer cells, and viruses. White blood cells require about 50 times more vitamin C on the inside than the outside and sugar competes with vitamin C for entry into white blood cells.[2]

Sugars can also contribute to a condition known as candidiasis (overgrowth of yeasts known as *Candida albicans*). A diet rich in carbohydrates stimulates yeast growth. When you eat sweets and other simple carbs, you feed the yeast in your intestinal tract, which can cause them to multiply rapidly. Weight gain and a host of illnesses and adverse symptoms are attributed to candidiasis.

If you crave sweets, breads, potatoes, or any other form of carbs, fill out the Candida Questionnaire on page 101 to help determine if you have an overgrowth of yeast in your body. Unless you deal with yeasts, you may never be able to lose the weight you want. The late Dr. Robert C. Atkins said that about 20 percent of the people on the Atkins Diet would not be able to lose weight because of yeasts.[3]

Overconsumption of sugar can also lead to *insulin resistance* (see page 34), which contributes to weight gain and a host of physical ailments including autoimmune disorders such as arthritis and multiple sclerosis, some forms of cancer, candidiasis, celiac disease, chronic fatigue syndrome, depression, type 2 diabetes, digestive disorders, heart disease, hyperlipidemia, hypertension, infertility, obesity, panic and anxiety attacks, hypoglycemia, and polycystic ovarian syndrome.

Natural Sweeteners

There are only a few natural sweeteners that I recommend for The Coconut Diet, and in very small quantities. Keep in mind, however, that a sweet taste could possibly trigger an insulin response, because your body may be conditioned to produce excess insulin no matter what the sweetener of choice, and if it has been doing this for a while, you may be insulin resistant. Therefore, in the first three weeks of the diet you should avoid all sweeteners as much as possible to give your body a chance to restore insulin sensitivity. (Many of the sweetener definitions in this section and the Refined Sweeteners section have been adapted from *The Goldbecks' Guide to Good Food*, by Nikki and David Goldbeck.)[4]

THE LOWER-CARB NATURAL SWEETENERS

- *Birch sugar (xylitol)* is a sugar alcohol. The healthiest xylitol is derived from birch bark. It has fewer calories than sugar with about the same sweetness. It has not been shown to promote tooth decay, and it is metabolized slowly, which helps prevent the sugar "highs" and "lows" often experienced with other sweeteners. Keep in mind that not all xylitol may be derived from birch bark. Some is made from by-products of the wood pulp industry; this should be avoided. There's only one brand I can recommend. (See Resources.)
- *Sugar alcohols* such as *sorbitol, mannitol, malitol,* and *xylitol* are sugar alcohols that are derived from dextrose or glucose, or in the case of xylitol, from birch trees or by-products of the pulp industry. On gum and candy labels they are often termed "sugar free," but this is somewhat misleading because when broken down, they act similarly to other forms of sugar. None are free of calories, and only xylitol has been shown to not promote cavities. Sugar alcohols tend to ferment in the digestive tract, causing cramping and diarrhea.
- *Lo Han Guo* comes from the Chinese plant Lo Han Guo *Siraitia grosvenorii,* a perennial vine in the cucumber or melon family that

grows in China. Lo Han Guo fruits contain triterpene glycoside sweeteners known as mogrosides. When processed into a fine powder, this natural sweetener is soluble in water. It is about 300 times sweeter than sugar, so very little is needed to sweeten foods and beverages. It is also very low in calories. No adverse effects have been associated with Lo Han Guo. It can be found in most health food stores.

- *Stevia* is extracted from an herbal leaf of a plant that grows in South America. Like Lo Han Guo, it is about 200 to 300 times sweeter than sugar, so a small amount sweetens in comparison to sugar. It has virtually no calories. There is no evidence that it is harmful to the body in any way. The FDA does not allow it to be marketed as a sweetener; rather it is labeled as a nutritional supplement. Stevia comes in powdered or liquid form and can be found at most health food stores.

THE HIGH-CARB NATURAL SWEETENERS: NOT GOOD CHOICES FOR WEIGHT LOSS

The only advantage that natural high-carb sweeteners have over those that are processed is natural sweeteners contain some nutrients and boast the absence of chemicals like those used in the processing and refining of other sweeteners. But they are still sugar. Be aware that they will raise blood sugar and insulin and they will contribute to insulin resistance and weight gain. All these sweeteners, with the exception of honey, are about equal in carbs to white sugar; honey is slightly higher.

- *Brown rice syrup* is a naturally fermented sweetener in which enzymes convert carbohydrates to maltose. Maltose may be tolerated somewhat better than other natural sweeteners by people with blood sugar metabolism disorders. It is made from wholegrain brown rice (malt barley syrup from barley) and contains some B vitamins and minerals. The consistency is similar to honey, but it is less sweet and more delicate and subtle. It can be found in most health food stores.

> I had lost 17 pounds just before I started on virgin coconut oil and have effortlessly lost an additional 6 pounds since I started including virgin coconut oil in my diet. A few months before I also stopped eating sugar and reduced my overall carb intake. I'm sure that has helped immensely.
>
> —*Julia*

- *Date sugar* is made of ground, dehydrated dates. It has a higher fiber (pectin) content than many other sweeteners and some vitamins and minerals. It can be found at most health food stores.
- *Honey* (raw is best) is composed of simple sugars, and it is both sweeter and slightly higher in carbs and calories than white sugar. Thus when preparing recipes, you would use less honey than white sugar. Its composition, color, and flavor are as varied as the blossoms that feed the honeybees. Most *raw* honey has been lightly heated and filtered, and retains some of the enzymes and traces of vitamins and minerals. Most commercial honey has been highly processed, and therefore, is less nutritional. Raw honey is usually available in health food stores and from private growers.
- *Pure maple syrup* is made by boiling the sap of sugar maple trees. It is less sweet than honey but sweeter than brown rice syrup and malt barley syrup. It comes in different grades according to how long and at what temperature it is boiled. The purest maple syrup may be imported from Canada because some U.S. producers use formaldehyde pellets to keep tapholes open. Look for labels that indicate the syrup has no added salt, chemical preservatives, or defoamers.
- *Molasses* is a by-product of the sugarcane refining process. Blackstrap molasses has a strong, bittersweet taste while sweet molasses is sweeter than blackstrap, but less sweet than white sugar. Blackstrap molasses is the final excretion of sugarcane and has some calcium, iron, and other minerals. A more nutritious purchase is

unsulphured molasses, which is most readily found in health food stores.

- *Raw sugarcane* is the product that exists before the bleaching stages of making refined sugar. To prepare this sugar for market, it is steam-cleaned; it retains a fraction of the dark molasses produced in sugar refining. Raw sugar is not subjected to the same chemical whitening as white sugar. Raw sugar is marketed under the names Turbinado or Sucanat, which can be found at most health food stores.

REFINED SWEETENERS: POOR CHOICES FOR WEIGHT MANAGEMENT AND HEALTH

- *White sugar* refers to the pure white crystals that remain after sugarcane or beets are refined; the chemical name is sucrose. To produce white sugar, this product goes through a series of washings, filterings, and bleachings, and nutrients are stripped away. Since raw sugarcane is brown and sticky, most refineries use slaughterhouse bone ash as a filtering agent to remove the molasses and create a free-flowing sugar. This sugar has virtually no nutritional value. It is readily available and found in many commercial desserts and packaged foods and treats. It is known to cause cavities and a host of other health problems.
- *Brown sugar* is mostly white sugar flavored with molasses. Its brown color comes from a charcoal treatment that may introduce traces of carcinogenic impurities, resulting in a product that is more refined and possibly more harmful than white sugar.
- *Fructose* is the chemical name for one kind of sugar that occurs naturally in honey and ripe fruit. The connection between commercial fructose and natural fruit sugar is in name only, however. The product found most often in packaged foods and table sweeteners is not from fruit or honey. Powdered fructose is often extracted from sugarcane, beet sugar, or corn syrup. In processing, the sucrose molecule breaks down into two simple sugars—fructose and glucose. This makes fructose more processed than white sugar and a worse choice for health.

Calorically, fructose is equivalent to sugar, but it is sweeter, so less is needed. Though fructose is often recommended for diabetics because it doesn't affect blood sugar and insulin levels like sucrose, it actually is more likely to cause insulin resistance. Studies on animals and humans have shown that consumption of large amounts of fructose impairs the body's ability to handle glucose (blood sugar), which ultimately leads to hyperinsulinemia (elevated insulin levels) and insulin resistance. Dr. Meira Field says, "All fructose must be metabolized in the liver. [In studies] the livers of rats on a high-fructose diet looked like the livers of alcoholics, plugged with fat and cirrhotic."[5]

- *Corn syrup* and high-fructose corn syrup are highly refined sweeteners made from corn. Corn syrup is composed of dextrose and small amounts of fructose. It is considerably cheaper than sugar, which accounts for its popularity in processed food. Manufacturers make high-fructose corn syrup by converting some of the dextrose in corn syrup to fructose. This sweetener should be avoided.

- *Dextrose* is a powdered form of corn sweetener that is used widely by food processors. It is structurally similar and biologically identical to glucose. This sweetener should be avoided.

- *Table syrup (includes maple-flavored syrup, pancake syrup, and waffle syrup)* is often confused with pure maple syrup. These syrups can actually look and taste like maple syrup, but they are made from a blend of sweeteners with emulsifiers, stabilizers, salt, viscosity adjusting agents, acidifiers, alkalizers or buffers, defoaming agents, artificial flavors and colors, additives, chemical preservatives, and fats and oils, as desired by the manufacturer. All these additives are not healthful and contribute to the body's burden of toxicity. This type of syrup should be avoided completely, even after you have achieved your weight loss goals.

Artificial Sweeteners: Avoid These Fakes

There is a great deal of controversy over sugar substitutes. I've placed them in the "completely avoid" category because of negative reports about some of them and the fact that the body doesn't recognize any of them because they are foreign substances that have undergone molecular changes. Such substances are not found in nature and have produced negative results for many people. That's why they don't have calorie counts; the body doesn't know what to do with them.

Miryam Ehrlich Williamson, author of *Blood Sugar Blues,* says she knows of people "who were unable to lose weight, and some who actually gained, on a low-carbohydrate diet that included liberal use of sugar substitutes." Her hunch is that some people are conditioned to pump insulin whenever they taste something sweet, just as Pavlov's dog learned to salivate when it heard a bell.[6]

Blood sugar and insulin spikes aren't the only concern with these sweeteners. Artificial sweeteners were first introduced decades ago as saccharin, which is 300 times sweeter than sugar. It was later packaged under the brand name Sweet 'n Low and in 1977 it was found to cause bladder cancer in lab animals. Because of public outcry it was not banned; it now comes with a cancer-warning label.

The most widely used artificial sweetener today is aspartame, popularly known as Equal or NutraSweet. Though more research may need to be done, current data collected from thousands of reports indicate that aspartame may contribute to headaches, mood changes, neurological disorders, seizures, and brain tumors.[7] And if that's not enough of a deterrent, it doesn't appear to help with weight loss either. A study published in the *International Journal of Obesity* monitored 14 women on weight loss diets who were given drinks of aspartame-sweetened lemonade, sucrose-sweetened lemonade, and carbonated mineral water on three separate days. The women ate significantly more food when they drank the aspartame-sweetened beverages.[8]

One of the latest and most popular artificial sweeteners is sucralose—sold under the brand name Splenda. To make sucralose, three components of a sugar molecule are replaced with three chlorine components. It is hundreds of times sweeter than sugar and has no calories; the body doesn't recognize it or know what to do with it because of the molecular changes.

Another new substitute is Sweet One. This sweetener is derived

THE WORST CARBS

- Alcohol: wine, beer, hard liquor
- Chips and crackers made with refined flour
- Breads, rolls, biscuits, bagels, buns, and pizza dough made with refined flour
- Most muffins
- Pasta made with refined flour
- White potatoes
- Cookies
- Cakes, pastries, and other baked goods
- Candy
- White rice, rice cakes, and puffed rice cereal

from vinegar and has a similar molecular structure as saccharin with no caloric value.

It's too soon to know what unhealthy effects these new sweeteners may produce in the body or if they cause people to eat more food. But why be a human test case with sugar substitutes the body can't recognize or use? It appears that every other artificial sweetener that has been studied has had adverse effects on the body; it's wise to stick with natural sweeteners the body can recognize.

THE GLYCEMIC RESPONSE

In 1981 David Jenkins developed the glycemic index to measure the rise in blood glucose after consumption of a particular food. This index shows the rate at which carbohydrates break down to glucose in the bloodstream. Test subjects are given a specified amount (50 grams) of carbohydrate in a test food and then their blood glucose is measured over a period of time to see how it is affected. The blood sugar response is compared with a standard food, usually white bread, and a rating is given to determine how blood sugar is affected.[9]

Though the glycemic index provides some insights as to how foods react in our bodies, there are numerous inconsistencies in connecting this index with the actual physical response. Due to this fact, some researchers have been attempting to determine the relative glucose area (RGA) of foods, which explains some of the inconsistencies in the glycemic index.[10]

Different carbohydrates take different pathways in the body after digestion. For example, some starchy foods are bound by an outer layer of very complex starches like the legumes (beans, lentils, split peas), which increases the time it takes for them to be digested. So even though legumes are relatively high in carbohydrates, they have a lower glycemic response because of their complex encasing.

Carrots are another example of glycemic inconsistency. If a person consumes 50 grams of carrots, which are required for the test, they've eaten about five cups of carrots. Not many persons would eat that many carrots. And even in that high quantity, carrots are still in the low glycemic category, just a little higher than many other vegetables.

There is also the antioxidant potential of foods to consider, meaning the amount of antioxidant nutrients a food contains, like beta carotene and vitamin C, that are abundant in many fruits and vegetables. Carrots and beets (very rich in beta-carotene) are often targeted as vegetables we should toss out with the potato chips, yet carrots are in the low glycemic category and beets are moderate. In Chinese culture, carrots are often used as cooling medicine.[11]

Carrots, beets, and other brightly colored vegetables are especially important to include in the diet to prevent disease. Today, many health professionals and diet doctors suggest eliminating carrots and beets from the diet because of their glycemic rating, but The Coconut Diet does not exclude them because of their high nutrient and fiber content.

The New Glucose Revolution: Complete Guide to Glycemic Index Values (Pub Group West) may be helpful for you to determine the foods that are higher in sugar. This guide offers the glycemic index value of most foods in a small book size that you can carry with you for quick reference.[12]

I have been on coconut oil for about two weeks. Instead of easing into it, I went gung ho and experienced a rapid detox. This is the first time in a *very long time* that I had no PMS symptoms! [Normally] I would have a huge craving for Coke, chocolate, and salt. I did not experience this at all. I had only one Coke. [When I drank it], it did not taste the same. My moodiness, cramps, and bloating [are gone]. I usually get a hormonal headache that sends me to bed. [which has] tormented me for over 20 years. This time, I had [only] a dull nagging ache that lasted just a day. I was amazed. The only change I made in my diet was adding coconut oil and cod liver oil. I really attribute this to the coconut oil as I have been consistent with it. I am really excited about this!

—*Judith*

The Coconut Diet eliminates the foods that are higher on the glycemic index and those foods that do not have fiber and turn to glucose rapidly. It eliminates the foods that aren't rich in nutrients and omits fruit for the first three weeks because of the higher sugar content and because many people suffer from yeast overgrowth, which fruit sugar promotes. This diet encourages foods that do not promote a rapid rise in insulin and, therefore, do not promote fat storage, and foods that are rich in fiber and thus slow down the release of sugar into the bloodstream.

WHAT CAUSES SUGAR CRAVINGS?

High-carb foods usually cause the pancreas to overcompensate by releasing too much insulin. This causes blood sugar to swing too low. You feel hungry, moody, and irritable. Other hormones are released, including cortisone and norepinephrine. Norepinephrine makes you nervous and stimulates the brain to crave more carbs. So

The past three days my sugar cravings have been gone. I actually didn't realize it until I was driving today and thought to myself, "I haven't had any sugar attacks in at least two days." Recently, the only thing I have done differently was to bump up the amount of virgin coconut oil I was taking. I was getting two to three tablespoons per day. Now I am adding three tablespoons directly to my morning smoothie (made with stevia, no sugar) and then getting some more [oil] with cooking and such. I have been doing this for about a week. The morning energy boost is awesome and I really feel good. My son was eating chocolate-covered raisins last night, which is normally a huge snack time for me. He passed the box to me and I ate a couple and then handed it back. It did nothing for me. I am so elated that maybe I can finally get the sugar out of my system and get my immune system back up to par. I would love for my recurrent yeast infections to be a thing of the past, too.

—*Michelle*

you eat a bowl of breakfast flakes, or a bagel, cookie, or bowl of ice cream. And your blood sugar goes up and then way down.

Sugar cravings can also be caused by a yeast overgrowth known as *Candida albicans*. This condition can sometimes cause uncontrollable urges to eat sweets (one of the preferred foods for yeast). If you suspect this might be you, fill in the Candida Questionnaire on page 101. Also, a chromium (trace mineral) deficiency can cause sugar cravings as can a protein deficiency.

Whatever the root cause, this cycle of carb cravings, blood sugar swings, and mood shifts leads to carbohydrate addiction, insulin resistance, and weight gain. This can be true for many individuals who find it difficult to lose weight. In many cases overweight individuals eat less food than normal weight individuals, but their choices are often simple carbohydrate foods due to carbohydrate cravings, or specifically sugar cravings.

THE TRUTH ABOUT INSULIN

Insulin is a powerful hormone. Primarily it pushes glucose out of the blood and into muscle, where it is converted into energy, and it shuttles nutrients into cells. It plays a critical role in blood sugar balance, weight management, and many other important health factors.

When blood sugar goes up, the pancreas releases insulin to deal with the sugar, but it often overreacts by releasing too much insulin. Then blood sugar goes down, often way down, and so more carbs are craved to bring it up again. And then the pancreas releases more insulin to deal with the carbs eaten—and on it goes.

Alcohol, pastries, candy, ice cream, pie, cake, and refined flour products such as bread, bagels, and pasta, as well as starches such as white potatoes and white rice rapidly break down to sugar and quickly enter the bloodstream where it causes insulin to spike. "It doesn't take much to cause your blood sugar to go up," says Ron Rosedale, M.D. He notes that one saltine cracker can take blood sugar to over 100, and in many people it can cause it to go over 150.[13]

I am an RN, [with a] bachelor's in nursing, master's in psych, and [am] finishing my doctorate in holistic health science. I have followed the path of diabetes through all the stages. I take 20–30 supplements a day, some to lower my blood sugar and others [for] antioxidants. Recently, I reluctantly went on Actos, which lowered my escalating blood sugar from 279 fasting and over 300–400 after a meal to 197 fasting and 200–300 after meals. Then I ran out [of Actos] and was unable to fill my prescription. (I am disabled from a lifting injury, [and] Medicare doesn't pay for Rx.) I upped my Vanadyl and [did] everything else I could think of to keep levels down, [but] to no avail. Bright and early this morning, after only one "dose" of the coconut oil, my fasting was 179. Absolutely no lie!

—*Cleora, RN, BSN*

When insulin becomes overabundant, the normal target cells in the muscles and liver will no longer recognize it. When this happens on a continual basis, a bunch of insulin floats around in the bloodstream all the time. When insulin becomes the dominant, active hormone, it triggers a hormone imbalance that sets the stage for weight gain, obesity, type 2 diabetes, and even cancer.

INSULIN RESISTANCE

Once glucose is in the blood, insulin carries it to the trillions of cells in the body. When you are more insulin sensitive, your body will do a much better job of shuttling glucose (blood sugar) and nutrients

I want to pass along a bit of my experience with regard to diabetes. I have been taking coconut oil for several months. I first started cooking with it and replacing the vegetable oils in my home. Then I started taking it by the spoonful—about two tablespoons daily. I was diagnosed as a type 2 diabetic in July of 2001 and immediately put on medication. I have been looking for a way to reverse this condition since diagnosed. I have found a world of info out there on various supplements and diet, but not from my doctor, who just said, "Welcome to the club!" and told me to take my meds. He also sent me to a nutritionist to take diabetic classes.

Bottom line is this: I have been able to work with my doctor to slowly remove myself from the medication and control my blood sugar with diet, supplements, and coconut oil. I am now off the medication. I do still check my blood sugar levels once or twice daily, and they are as good as, usually better than, when I was taking the drugs.

I hope this may help someone. God bless all.

—*Sharon*

into your cells. The "open doors" of your cells allow this fuel in where it is used for energy. How easily glucose is shuttled in means how sensitive your cells are to insulin.[14]

When your cells are not sensitive to insulin, insulin levels go up. Target cells will develop what is termed *insulin resistance,* which leads to hyperinsulinemia. When your cells are insulin resistant, your body must contend with extra "free roaming" glucose that can't get into your cells. Some of this will be stored as fat and lead to weight gain. Without insulin sensitivity, you may struggle with your weight continually over a lifetime.[15]

In light of these facts, it is vitally important to stick faithfully with a low-refined-carb diet, not only to facilitate weight loss, but also to prevent premature aging and disease. To assess your sensitivity, see the Insulin Resistance Quiz, page 39.

HOW TO IMPROVE
INSULIN SENSITIVITY

Insulin sensitivity can be restored to a healthful state, which not only results in weight loss, but also in improved health. The right diet like The Coconut Diet is key to improving insulin sensitivity. There's no magic bullet involved—it's good choices made daily that will make all the difference. Here's what you can do:

- *Avoid sweets* and other simple carbohydrates (refined grains, alcohol, and starches); this is one of the most important steps you can take.
- *Avoid artificial sweeteners* and nicotine as they cause an increase in insulin. A diet soda or an artificial sweetener in your coffee, even though it has no calories, sends confusing signals to your body. Though these artificial sweeteners do not cause blood sugar levels to rise, they can cause insulin levels to increase, which can lead to low blood sugar, weakness, hunger, and ultimately insulin resistance.[16] You may think that you are serving your weight loss goals by choosing artificial, noncalorie sweeteners, but in fact, you can

be setting yourself up for a lifelong struggle with weight management due to insulin resistance and an increased appetite caused by the artificial sweeteners.

- *Cut back on coffee.* Drinking just two cups of coffee per day has been shown to increase levels of the stress hormone cortisol. When this hormone is elevated, it can cause adverse effects on the immune system, brain cells, sugar metabolism (which includes setting you up for insulin resistance), and weight gain. Coffee drinking has been reported to cause increased body fat, often around the midsection, due to insulin and cortisol elevation. (Stress also causes cortisol to go up.) Clinical studies show that when coffee intake is reduced, body fat goes down.[17] If you just can't give up that cup of java, make sure you have no more than one cup a day. The rest of the day, try drinking tea—either herbal or green tea—water, sparkling mineral water, and some fresh vegetable juice. (Green tea has some caffeine; about one-third that of coffee.)

- *Green tea can help you lose weight.* When tea was substituted for coffee, especially green tea, it had the opposite effect—it helped people lose weight.[18] Avoid green tea (and all other sources of caffeine) if you are hypothyroid, have adrenal stress, or are hypoglycemic; green tea does contain caffeine, which should be omitted until these conditions are corrected.

- *Increase your intake of essential fatty acids.* You can increase cell receptor activity by increasing the fluidity of cell membranes. Omega-3 fatty acids, especially docosahexaenoic acid (DHA) actually make cell membranes more fluid. Essential fatty acids also help to lower levels of "stress chemicals" such as cortisol and norepinephrine. This may account, in part, for one weight loss study's success with omega-3s, published in the *American Journal of Clinical Nutrition,* which showed the best weight loss results, along with reduction of glucose and insulin, in the group that ate one meal of fish each day.[19]

- *Learn stress reduction techniques* and how to manage stress effectively. This can definitely help improve insulin resistance. High levels of stress activate the "fight or flight" response, which

SIX STEPS TO IMPROVING BLOOD SUGAR BALANCE AND INSULIN SENSITIVITY

1. Follow The Coconut Diet. The meal plans and recipes in this book are designed to help you improve your blood sugar balance and improve insulin sensitivity.
2. Eat only healthy fats and oils. Healthful oils help promote insulin sensitivity. This is one more reason I recommend only virgin coconut oil, extra virgin olive oil, and essential fatty acids (the omega-3s), which are found in coldwater fish such as salmon and sardines, fish oils such as cod liver oil (rich in EPA [eicosapentaenoic acid] and DHA), flaxseeds, and evening primrose oil or black currant oil.
3. Eat only complex carbohydrates; avoid simple carbs. Vegetables, legumes, whole grains, and fruit are rich in fiber; they release their sugars more slowly into the bloodstream. Simple carbohydrates such as sugar (all sweets), refined flour products, and starches like white potatoes and white rice, break down rapidly into glucose and cause blood sugar to rise. They should be avoided as part of a healthy lifestyle.
4. Eat a moderate amount of lean protein. Protein stimulates the release of glucagon, a hormone that mobilizes fat stores into energy, and it plays an important part in blood sugar stability. Choose naturally raised, organically fed animal products. Such animals yield healthier, leaner proteins. But eat protein moderately. Overconsumption of protein can cause an increase in uric acid and taxes the kidneys.
5. Exercise on a regular basis. Aerobic exercise and strength training help increase insulin sensitivity.
6. Drink green or herbal tea, avoid coffee, and drink 8–10 glasses of water each day.

stimulates epinephrine production. Epinephrine causes the liver and muscles to convert glucose from its reserved state as glycogen to its active sugar form. Insulin rises to control glucose and increased insulin levels signal fat storage. This is one reason why some stressed individuals cannot lose weight regardless of how strict they are with their food choices. Relaxation techniques such as massage, hydrotherapy, aromatherapy, and prayer can improve insulin sensitivity and fat loss.[20]

Now that you know which carbs are good and which ones are bad, you can make wise choices the rest of your life that will encourage healthy blood sugar balance. In the next chapter, you'll learn the truth about fats and oils. If you were surprised by some of the information about carbs in this chapter, then you'll probably be amazed at how misinformed our culture has been about fats. Saturated fats have gotten a bad rap for no good reason. And, a lot of misinformation about these fats has been popularized in mainstream media. Chapter 3, "The Big Fat Misconception," presents the lowdown on fats and oils. It is quite possible that your entire manner of preparing food will never be the same after you finish this chapter. Best of all, you'll discover which fats make you fat and which ones help you trim your waistline.

INSULIN RESISTANCE QUIZ
HOW INSULIN RESISTANT ARE YOU?

Part 1

1. Do you spend more time than you'd like to worrying about your weight? (Score 1 for yes, 0 for no.) _____

2. Do you feel sleepy or fatigued an hour or two after eating? (Score 1 for yes, 0 for no.) _____

3. Do you experience anxiety or panic attacks? (Score 1 for yes, 0 for no.) _____

4. Score 1 point for every symptom you have from the list below:

   Abnormal triglycerides or cholesterol levels _____

   Binge eating, uncontrollable cravings _____

   Bloating or abdominal gas _____

   Chronic fatigue _____

   Chronic indigestions _____

   Depression that comes and goes _____

   Food/chemical allergies _____

   Gastrointestinal (digestive tract) problems _____

   Heart trouble (heart attack, congestive heart failure, etc.) _____

   Hypertension (high blood pressure) _____

   Inability to lose weight on a low-fat diet _____

   Infertility/irregular menstrual periods _____

   Mental confusion or "brain fog" _____

   Obesity (20 percent or more, over your ideal weight) _____

   Total, part 1 _____

Continued

Part 2

1. Measure your waist and hips. Divide your waist measurement
    by your hip measurement.

    Women: If the result is .8 or more, score 10 points _____

    Men: If the result is 1.0 or more, score 10 points _____

2. Give yourself 1 point for every blood relative who
    has diabetes.   _____

3. By how many pounds are you overweight?   _____

4. Give yourself 1 point for every time you've gone
    on a diet.   _____

                    Total, part 2   _____

                    Total, parts 1 and 2   _____

Interpreting the Results

Part 1: The maximum possible score is 20. The higher your score,
the greater the likelihood that you will benefit from the lifestyle
changes outlined in this book.

Part 2: There is no maximum score. If you recorded a 10 in
answer to the first question, you are by definition insulin resistant. If you scored the first question as 0 but your total in part 2
is 15 or more, you have reason to be concerned.

A total for both parts of 35 or more tells you it's time to take
action.

Chapter 3

The Big Fat Misconception

For decades we have been told to cut back on the fats in our diet if we want to maintain a healthy weight and prevent heart disease. Marketers of low-fat foods have championed this concept. But according to the U.S. Centers for Disease Control (CDC) statistics, the results have not been what we were promised. In 1999–2000, an estimated 30 percent of U.S. adults aged 20 years and older—that's nearly 59 million people—were obese, defined as having a body mass index (BMI) of 30 or more, and 64 percent of U.S. adults aged 20 years and older were either overweight or obese, defined as having a BMI of 25 or more.[1] (The BMI is a measuring system that determines obesity based on body-fat content rather than weight.) That accounts for almost two-thirds of the U.S. adult population being classified as overweight. And heart disease is still the number one killer of Americans.

Health and Human Services Secretary Tommy G. Thompson said, "We've seen virtually a doubling in the number of obese persons over the past two decades and this has profound health implications. Obesity increases a person's risk for a number of serious conditions, including diabetes, heart disease, stroke, high blood pressure, and some types of cancer."[2]

Obviously, low-fat diets have not helped Americans lose weight. Isn't it time to stop this insanity about fat? Fat is not the substance making most of us overweight. Not that overeating fats wouldn't put weight on, but the major culprit for most people is refined carbohydrates—foods like sugar, potato chips, soda pop, pasta, pizza, breads, and other products made with refined grains. These types of foods are without doubt the major reason Americans are fat. And it's no wonder! They are a big part of the typical American diet.

Consumers have heard for years that they should avoid fat as much as possible. Some people have been on a torturous low-fat regimen, trying to avoid all fat in their diet. Now folks are learning about the dangers of low-fat diets. Health professionals have had a chance to observe the results of years of eating low-fat and no-fat diets— results that have been very detrimental to our health. We need good fats, especially the essential fatty acids, to stay healthy. And we need a certain amount of fat in our diet to prevent overeating.

We are also learning that the saturated fat scare has turned out to be—a "big fat lie"! Gary Taubes wrote a startling article in the *New York Times* magazine, July 7, 2002, titled "What If It's All Been a Big Fat Lie?" In it he stated:

The cause of obesity [is] precisely those refined carbohydrates at the base of the famous Food Guide Pyramid—the pasta, rice and bread—that we are told should be the staple of our healthy, low-fat diet, and then add on the sugar or corn syrup in the soft drinks, fruit juices, and sports drinks that we have taken to consuming in quantity if for no other reason than that they are fat free and so appear intrinsically healthy. While the low-fat-is-good-health dogma represents reality as we have come to know it, and the government has spent hundreds of millions of dollars in research trying to prove its worth, the low-carbohydrate message has been relegated to the realm of unscientific fantasy.

Over the past five years, however, there has been a subtle shift in the scientific consensus. Now a small but growing minority of establishment researchers have come to take seriously what the low-carb-diet doctors have been saying all along. Walter Willett, chairman of the department of nutrition at the Harvard School of Public Health, may be the most visible proponent of testing this heretic hypothesis. Willett is the de facto spokesman of the longest-running, most comprehensive diet and health studies ever performed, which have already cost upward of $100 million and include data on nearly 300,000 individuals. "Those data," says Willett, "clearly contradict the low-fat-is-good-health message and the idea that all fat is bad for you; the exclusive focus on adverse effects of fat may have contributed to the obesity epidemic."[3]

FATS THAT HEAL

Fats have always been a part of human nutrition, until the late twentieth century that is, and they were even recommended in days of yore for treating serious medical conditions.

Rex Russell, M.D., writes: "It was 1944, and World War II was roaring. A young mother was wasting away with an infection diagnosed as tuberculosis. Antibiotics were unavailable. Her doctor prescribed (1) isolation, (2) bed rest, (3) exercise (eventually), and (4) *a diet high in fat*. Surprising, but true! High-fat diets were often the recommended protocol by the medical profession during those years. Before you scoff, you might want to know that this lady recovered. She is my mother, and she has stayed on this diet through the years. Presently she is enjoying her great-grandchildren."[4]

While the experts claimed, "fats are good," prior to World War II, consumers have heard just the opposite in recent years. What actually constituted a "high-fat" diet prior to the late 1940s was mostly butter, cream, eggs, lard, and beef tallow. Today, just mentioning some of these fats makes many people gasp, but they made up the typical diet of yesteryear. Margarines, which were introduced in the U.S. in 1871, were butter substitutes made with animal fats such as lard and beef tallow or the saturated vegetable oils from coconut oil and palm oils, with yellow dye added to make them look like butter. They were much healthier than the margarine today made of hydrogenated or partially hydrogenated vegetable oil that contains transfatty acids.

Today, saturated fats are considered by many people to be the

I've been taking about one to two tablespoons of virgin coconut oil per day for about four months now. I definitely notice a difference in my energy. It's steady through the day—no longer have the surges of ups and downs, especially that sleepy feeling after a meal.

—*Marty*

I am 52 years old and I am keeping up with my visiting grandsons (6 and 8 years old) as if I am 30-something. I have lost 10 pounds in about five weeks and have 10 more to go. My dry eyes are gone along with the aches and pains of arthritis, Sjogren's, osteoporosis, and fibromyalgia. I feel like the combination of my good diet, the virgin coconut oil, and exercise is the key to my success.

—*Sharon*

worst fats one can consume. However, drastically reducing saturated fats from the modern diet has not solved the nation's health problems. Statistics show that obesity rates are at an all-time high as is heart disease, cancer, diabetes, and stroke. The low-fat advice is losing credibility. And, surprisingly, people on a high-fat diet using coconut oil are discovering that many of their ailments as well as excess weight are disappearing and cholesterol and triglycerides are lowering.

ABOUT FATS AND OILS

Fats and oils are technically known as "lipids." If a lipid is liquid at room temperature, it is called *oil*. If it is solid, it is called *fat*. Fats can be found in many food sources in nature: animal products (butter, cream, tallow, and lard), fish (fish oil), vegetables and fruits (olive, avocado, corn), nuts (walnut, coconut, macadamia nut), seeds (grape seed, sesame seed), legumes (peanut, soybean), and whole grains (wheat, rice, rye). Grains must contain all of their components, which we call *whole grains,* to benefit from all the oils present. A diet rich in natural whole foods will be a high-fat diet. It is virtually impossible to eliminate fats from our food unless we refine them. Fats are an essential part of life. Without them, we could not survive.

Four vitamins—A, D, E, and K—are fat-soluble vitamins, meaning they are soluble in fat and fat transports them in our body. When fat is removed from a food, many of the fat-soluble vitamins and other healthful compounds are also removed and the carrier of fat-soluble vitamins is unavailable.

Fat also gives rich flavor to food. It adds satiety to a meal—a feeling of having had enough to eat. Fat-free and low-fat foods are one of the reasons some people overeat carbohydrates, which really packs on the pounds. These people just don't feel as if they've had enough to eat many times, even when the volume has been more than ample.

One very good reason to add coconut oil to your weight loss plan is that it satisfies hunger better than any other fat, as well as most other types of food. For this reason, many people say they feel full eating less food at a meal and can go for longer periods of time without getting hungry. This helps prevent unnecessary snacking.

I am marveling over and over about how this coconut oil is working! By the time I finished my first quart of virgin coconut oil, I could tell my hypoglycemic hunger cravings were subsiding, and my taste for coffee and chocolate was changing. I feel like a "born-again believer."

—*Beverly*

I have been on virgin coconut oil for the past two months (four tablespoons daily) and feel better than I have in a long time! My energy levels are up and my weight is down. I am never hungry anymore, and have incorporated a daily exercise routine. I have lost 20 pounds.

—*Paula*

THE BENEFITS OF SATURATED FATS

Saturated fats have not only been a major part of our forefathers' diets, they have been a big part of the diets of traditional cultures. Tropical diets, for example, obtain much of their fats from coconut and palm oils, which are rich in saturated fats. As discussed in chapter 1, these cultures have not had the obesity problems that we see today in American culture, even though they've had a diet high in saturated fats.

Saturated fats have a long history of use in traditional cultures because they are very stable fats that do not easily oxidize (turn rancid). Virgin coconut oil, for example, will not turn rancid at room temperature in the tropics for up to two years. Conversely, the refined oils that many Americans use are very unstable and turn rancid (oxidize) quickly. Heating polyunsaturated fatty acids (PaFAs) tends to polymerize these oils (form chemical compounds known as polymers). Oxidized oils are very toxic to the body and they can cause widespread free-radical damage.

In addition to their shelf stability, saturated fats have many important roles in the body's chemistry: For example:

- Saturated fatty acids constitute at least 50 percent of cell membranes. They give cells necessary firmness and integrity.
- Saturated fats play a vital role in the health of bones. For example, at least 50 percent of dietary fats need to be saturated for calcium to be effectively incorporated into the skeletal structure.[5]
- Saturated fats lower Lp(a), a substance in the blood that indicates proneness to heart disease.[6]
- Saturated fats protect the liver from the toxic effects of alcohol and certain drugs.[7]
- Saturated fats enhance the immune system.[8]
- Saturated fats are needed for the proper utilization of essential fatty acids. Elongated omega-3 fatty acids are better retained in the tissues when the diet is rich in saturated fats.[9]
- Saturated 18-carbon stearic acid and 16-carbon palmitic acid are the preferred foods for the heart: the fat around the heart

muscle is highly saturated.[10] The heart draws on this reserve of fat in times of stress.

TOXIC OILS

Walk into any major grocery store or retail food chain and visit the cooking oil section—you will not find much in the form of saturated fats such as coconut or palm oils. Oils, known as *polyunsaturated oils,* have replaced saturated fats in modern cooking.

Unfortunately, polyunsaturated oils are not stable; they are very prone to oxidation. Modern commercial oils are a recent addition to the diet. After World War II, manufacturers developed a process to make them more shelf stable. Hydrogenating, or partially hydrogenating these oils also makes them more solid (mimicking saturated fats) and useful for baking and deep-frying.

The most common polyunsaturated oils commercially processed in the United States are soy, corn, cottonseed, rapeseed, and safflower; 90 percent of all margarines are made from soy oil and are loaded with toxic fatty acids. Research shows that the hydrogenation of these polyunsaturated oils creates a whole new subclass of fats called *trans-fatty acids.* These trans fats are not found in any appreciable amounts in nature and are very toxic. Studies are now showing that trans-fatty acids are linked to cardiovascular disease, diabetes, and cancer.

In January 2004, Denmark became the first country in the world to ban the manufacture of trans-fatty acids in its foods.[11] In Europe, the consumption of trans-fatty acids is decreasing. In the United States, the FDA is requiring all food manufacturers to list trans-fatty acids on the nutrition panel of their labels by the year 2006. The FDA website gives the following warning:

On July 9, 2003, FDA issued a regulation requiring manufacturers to list trans-fatty acids, or trans fat, on the Nutrition Facts panel of foods and some dietary supplements. With this rule, consumers have more information to make healthier food choices that could lower their consumption of trans fat as part of a heart-healthy diet. Scientific reports have confirmed the relationship between trans fat and an increased risk of coronary heart disease. Food manufacturers have until January 1, 2006, to list trans fat on the nutrition label. FDA estimates that by three years after that date, trans fat labeling will have prevented from 600 to 1,200 cases of coronary heart disease and 250 to 500 deaths each year.[12]

WHICH FATS MAKE US FAT?

The fatty acid chains in polyunsaturated oils are predominantly long-chain fatty acids (LCTs) while the fatty acid chains in coconut oil are mostly medium-chain fatty acids (MCTs). The scientific community has known for a long time that LCTs tend to produce fat in the body, while MCTs promote weight loss. People in the animal feed business have known this truth for quite some time as well. If you feed animals vegetable oils, they put on weight and produce more meat. If you feed them coconut oil, they will be very lean and active.

In a study published in the *American Journal of Clinical Nutrition*, for example, rats were fed MCTs and LCTs for six weeks. At the end of six weeks the rats were killed and dissected, and the total dissectible fat and fat cell size and number were determined. MCT-fed rats gained 15 percent less weight than LCT-fed controls. Their conclusion was that "overfeeding MCT diets results in decreased body fat related to increased metabolic rate and thermogenesis."[13]

Polyunsaturated oils can also contribute to weight gain by suppressing thyroid function, causing a lower metabolic rate that leads to packing on the pounds.

Dr. Ray Peat says:

Linoleic and linolenic acids, the "essential fatty acids," and other polyunsaturated fatty acids, which are now fed to pigs to fatten them, in the form of corn and soybeans, cause the animals' fat to be chemically equivalent to vegetable oil. In the

I have added coconut oil to my weight loss program, which is basically low carb, moderate protein, and reasonably high fat. I used this type of diet a few years ago and lost weight, but I "fell off the wagon" and put the weight back on. The major difference this time is that I have replaced all vegetable oils (corn, soy, canola, and so forth) with coconut oil and olive oil. When I eat a meal that has very lean protein, I take extra coconut oil. I have lost 58 pounds since December [that's in just eight months] with no exercise beyond a couple of walks per week. One positive side effect is that my resting heart rate has gone from 79 to 59.

I'm never hungry. In fact, I have to eat more than I feel like eating. Often times I could skip a meal, but I don't do it because I don't want my body to go into a starvation mode.

Perhaps the best part is that a lot of people are telling me I look younger.

—*Chuck*

late 1940s, chemical toxins were used to suppress the thyroid function of pigs, to make them get fatter while consuming less food. When that was found to be carcinogenic, it was then found that corn and soybeans had the same anti-thyroid effect, causing the animals to be fattened at low cost. The animals' fat becomes chemically similar to the fats in their food, causing it to be equally toxic, and equally fattening.[14]

THE SLIMMING FATS

Coconut oil is nature's richest source of MCTs, which increase metabolic rate and leads to weight loss. MCTs promote what is called *thermogenesis*. Thermogenesis increases the body's metabolism, producing energy. Many studies in the scientific literature support this.

In 1989 a study was completed in the Department of Pediatrics, Vanderbilt University, Nashville, Tennessee. Ten male volunteers (ages 22 to 44) were overfed (150 percent of estimated energy requirement) liquid formula diets containing 40 percent fat as either MCTs or LCTs. Each patient was studied for one week on each diet in a double-blind, crossover design. The researchers noted the following: "Our results demonstrate that excess dietary energy as MCT stimulates thermogenesis to a greater degree than does excess energy as LCT. This increased energy expenditure, most likely due to lipogenesis [formation of fatty acids] in the liver, provides evidence that excess energy derived from MCT is stored with a lesser efficiency than is excess energy derived from dietary LCT."[15]

In another study recently conducted at the School of Dietetics and Human Nutrition, McGill University, Ste-Anne-de-Bellevue, Quebec, Canada, the effects of diets rich in MCTs or LCTs on body composition, energy expenditure, substrate oxidation, subjective appetite, and ad libitum energy intake in overweight men was documented. Twenty-four healthy, overweight men with body mass indexes between 25 and 31 kg/m^2 consumed diets rich in MCT or LCT for 28 days, each in a crossover randomized controlled trial. The researchers concluded: "Consumption of a diet rich in MCTs results in greater loss of AT [adipose tissue] compared with LCTs, perhaps due to increased energy expenditure and fat oxidation observed with MCT intake. Thus, MCTs may be considered as agents that aid in the prevention of obesity or potentially stimulate weight loss."[16]

One "slimming fat" is a little known fatty acid called conjugated linoleic acid (CLA) found almost exclusively in ruminant animals and dairy fats. Research has shown that CLA tends to normalize body fat deposition. Without CLA, dietary fat tends to be stored in fat cells. Because CLA is negligible in most American diets, we can have trouble controlling our weight. The body cannot produce CLA; it must get it from food, the primary sources being beef and dairy products.

Americans do tend to eat a lot of meat products, so why are our CLA levels so low? People who study such things have found that the CLA content of these foods, if produced in the United States, is low. CLA count started falling around 1950, about the same time

I lost 17 pounds taking coconut oil. I did nothing else but add it to my skillet for dinner on some, but not all, nights and maybe in a few other experimental recipes.

—*Malikah*

that farmers began feeding cattle and dairy cows in feedlots, rather than allowing them to graze in pastures. Eating grass is what produces CLA in dairy cows and cattle.

We can, however, make CLA from the *trans*-vaccenic acid that comes from milk fat.[17] But most of us don't eat much butter, cheese, or cream. And that's a good idea because most of the animals in this country are not organically raised; indeed, they are injected with or fed antibiotics and growth hormones and pesticide-sprayed food. Toxins tend to be stored in the fat more than the muscle, and therefore, eating a lot of animal fat from factory farm–raised animals isn't the best idea.

In light of these facts, it is best to purchase grass-fed beef that has been raised organically (not injected with hormones and antibiotics), and to purchase dairy products from cows that are grass-fed and raised organically.

Best of all, you can include one of the most effective slimming fats, virgin coconut oil, into your daily diet and watch the pounds melt away.

MORE SCIENTIFIC EVIDENCE ON THE WEIGHT LOSS EFFECTS OF MCTS

Scientific studies have reported that the fatty acids from MCTs are not easily converted into stored triglycerides and that MCTs are not readily used by the body to make larger fat molecules.[18] One animal feeding study evaluated body weight and fat storage for three different diets—a low-fat diet, a high-fat diet containing LCTs, and a high-fat diet containing MCTs. All animals were fed the selected diets for 44 days. At the end of that time, the low-fat diet group had stored an average of 0.47 grams of fat per day; the LCT group stored 0.48 grams per day, while the MCT group deposited only 0.19 grams of fat per day—a 60 percent reduction in the amount of fat stored. The authors concluded: "the change from a low-fat diet to a MCT diet is attended by a decrease in the body weight gain."[19]

This study points out two important facts: First, when MCTs are substituted for LCTs in the diet, the body is much less inclined to store fat. Second, when we eat sensibly, a diet containing MCTs is more effective than a low-fat diet at decreasing stored fat.

In a human study, researchers compared the metabolic effects of 400-calorie meals of MCTs and LCTs by measuring metabolic rates prior to and six hours following the test meals. The results showed that the MCT-containing meals caused an average 12 percent increase in basal metabolic rate as compared with a 4 percent increase with the LCT-containing meal. The authors concluded that replacing dietary fats with MCTs could "over long periods of time produce weight loss even in the absence of reduced [caloric] intake."[20]

ESSENTIAL FATTY ACIDS

Two fatty acids are considered essential to human health and cannot be formed in the body—omega-3 (alpha-linolenic acid) and omega-6 (linoleic) fatty acids; they must be supplied through diet. Because it is believed that our body cannot manufacture these fatty acids, they are considered essential fatty acids (EFAs).

Although these fatty acids are essential, our bodies do not need a lot of them. It is believed we need only about 2 to 3 percent of our caloric intake from omega-6 fatty acids and about 0.5 to 1.5 percent of our caloric intake from omega-3 fatty acids. Omega-6 fatty acids are primarily found in foods such as corn, soybeans, sunflower seeds, and cottonseeds. Omega-3 fatty acids are found primarily in flax and hemp seeds, fish, and fish oils.

Because of the amount of polyunsaturated oils in a contemporary diet, most people consume a much higher ratio of omega-6 to omega-3 fatty acids. In addition, research shows that a proper amount of saturated fat is needed in the diet to enable the body to adequately utilize omega-3 fatty acids.[21] Many people are considered to be deficient in omega-3 fatty acids, leading to potential health problems such as sleep disorders, depression, memory problems, weight gain, dry hair and skin, hair loss, brittle fingernails, allergies, poor concentration, arthritis, and fatigue.

One of the best ways to increase intake of omega-3 fatty acids is by supplementing the diet with a good brand of cod liver oil. (Look for cod liver oil that comes from cod caught in the waters around Iceland or Norway.) Fish oil provides two essential fatty acids found in the omega-3 family called EPA (eicosapentaenoic acid) and DHA (docosahexaenoic acid), which are not found in plant sources. Some studies have linked EPA and DHA to certain health benefits, such as improved vision and mental awareness, as well as prevention of diseases like cancer and heart disease. Cod liver oil is also high in vitamin D, a nutrient many people are lacking, especially during the long winter months when there is little exposure to sunlight. It is also a good source of vitamin A, which may be particularly helpful for people with a hypothyroid condition.

CHOLESTEROL AND SATURATED FATS

There is a question as to whether cholesterol causes heart disease. Uffe Ravnskov, M.D., Ph.D. (author of *The Cholesterol Myths*); Malcom Kendrick, M.D.; Mary Enig, Ph.D.; George Mann, M.D.; Sc.D.; and many other top researchers have written extensively on the flaws of the "high cholesterol causing heart disease" theory.

More than 60 percent of all heart attacks occur in people with normal cholesterol levels. The majority of people with high cholesterol levels never have heart attacks.

Looking beyond cholesterol as a cause, researchers are now focusing on the following contributors to heart disease: (1) damaged fats—particularly trans fats, (2) high blood pressure, (3) inflammation, (4) blood clots, (5) the use of oils high in omega-6 fatty acids (polyunsaturated oils), and (6) high levels of homocysteine. The American Heart Association has discovered that people with heart disease all have one thing in common—inflammation.[22]

Coconut oil and saturated fats have been implicated for many years as a cause of increased cholesterol levels. People often ask whether coconut oil will raise their cholesterol levels.

In an article published in the *Indian Coconut Journal,* September 1995, Dr. Mary Enig stated, "The problems for coconut oil started four decades ago when researchers fed animals hydrogenated coconut oil that was purposely altered to make it completely devoid of any essential fatty acids. The animals fed the hydrogenated coconut oil (as the only fat source) naturally became essential fatty acid deficient; their serum cholesterol increased. Diets that cause an essential fatty acid deficiency always produce an increase in serum cholesterol levels as well as an increase in the atherosclerotic indices. The same effect has also been seen when other highly hydrogenated oils such as cottonseed, soybean, or corn oils have been fed; so it is clearly a function of the hydrogenated products, either because the oil is essential fatty acid (EFA) deficient or because of trans-fatty acids."[23]

Studies show that coconut oil actually increases (good) HDL cholesterol. When measurements of serum cholesterol (cholesterol levels in the blood) were first done, only the total of both good (HDL) and bad (LDL) cholesterol were read. Now that testing has become more sophisticated, researchers look more at the balance of these two types of cholesterol. They note whether a substance raises cholesterol levels of HDL or LDL levels. In some cases, certain foods lower total cholesterol, but only by lowering good HDL cholesterol, while at the same time actually raising levels of the bad LDL cholesterol.

In studies where animals were fed unprocessed coconut oil, Enig says: "Hostmark et al. (1980) compared the effects of diets containing 10 percent coconut oil and 10 percent sunflower oil on lipoprotein distribution in male Wistar rats. Coconut oil feeding produced

I just got tested after taking virgin coconut oil and my cholesterol is slightly down, but my triglycerides are way down—from 192 to 135.

—*Sandy*

I use virgin coconut oil, olive oil, and butter in my cooking and add extra virgin coconut oil to my smoothies, and [I also eat coconut oil] just by the tablespoon. My total cholesterol went down over 100 points; HDL and LDL were great! My coworkers could not believe I was eating so much fat and watching my cholesterol levels go down. I had to take a fasting [blood] test to prove it to them. I have lost 18 pounds in three months. I have learned a new way of life and it's easy. I'm healthier for it, too. I will never count calories again!

—*Laurel*

significantly lower levels ($p = 0.05$) of pre-beta-lipoproteins (VLDL) and significantly higher ($p = <0.01$) alpha-lipoproteins (HDL) relative to sunflower feeding." She also cited a study by Awad (1981) on Wistar rats fed a diet of either 14 percent (natural) coconut oil or 14 percent safflower oil. Commenting on that study, Dr. Enig says: "Total tissue cholesterol accumulation for animals on the safflower [oil] diet was six times greater than for animals fed the [unhydrogenated] coconut oil. A conclusion that can be drawn from some of the animal research is that feeding hydrogenated coconut oil devoid of essential fatty acids (EFA) potentiate the formation of atherosclerosis markers. It is of note that animals fed regular coconut oil have less cholesterol deposited in their livers and other parts of their bodies."[24]

A study published in 1973 in the *Journal Nutrition* reported that long-term feeding of medium-chain triglycerides (MCTs) at fairly high doses was able to reduce cholesterol levels.[25] And as stated earlier, coconut oil is nature's richest source of MCTs.

A study conducted by the Wynn Institute for Metabolic Research, London, examined the composition of human aortic plaques. This study found that the "artery clogging fats" in those who died from heart disease were composed of 26 percent saturated fat; the rest (74 percent) were polyunsaturated fatty acids, such as those found in vegetable oils commonly consumed in today's modern societies. Their conclusion was that "no associations were found with saturated fatty acids." These findings imply a direct influence of dietary polyunsaturated fatty acids on aortic plaque formation and suggest that current trends favoring increased intake of polyunsaturated fatty acids should be reconsidered.[26]

FACTORS THAT CONTRIBUTE TO HEART DISEASE

One of the solutions to heart disease is to reduce the causes of inflammation—one of the primary being *homocysteine*, a harmless acid-like waste product produced by the consumption of red meat and other protein foods. Homocysteine is normally broken down rapidly by some of the B vitamins, and so under normal circumstances it does not pose a problem. But when adequate amounts of B vitamins are lacking in the diet (which is the case for many people today), homocysteine will build up to dangerous levels and injure the delicate tissue of artery walls. Plaque is then formed at the site of the injury as the body attempts to heal the damage.[27]

Studies show that a high level of homocysteine is one of the most dangerous risk factors for heart disease. It increases a person's risk of heart attack by 300 percent. Including extra B vitamins in one's diet could do a lot to prevent heart disease. But many people do get adequate B vitamins in their diet and still have a deficiency. So what's the cause? An underactive thyroid gland can be at the root of the problem. When the thyroid gland malfunctions, absorption of B vitamins is inhibited, causing homocysteine levels to rise.

In 1976, Dr. Broda Barnes wrote a book titled *Solved: The Riddle of Heart Attacks*, which pointed to the connection between thyroid malfunction and heart attacks. His research was ignored by most of the medical community. But the Third National Health and Nutrition Examination Survey published findings in 2001 that confirmed this connection; they found a definite correlation between high cholesterol, elevated homocysteine, and hypothyroid.[28] It has been found that when thyroid function is corrected in patients, homocysteine levels normalize.

An underactive thyroid can cause a number of other health problems as well, such as Alzheimer's disease, depression, memory loss, and obesity. Symptoms can include weight gain, loss of sexual desire, cold hands and feet, a weak immune system, constipation, allergies, and much more. Many Americans suffer from an underactive thyroid gland. Yet the standard thyroid tests don't detect the problem for many people.

The problem is widespread because of significant agricultural changes over the past five decades that have created alarming mineral deficiencies in our food supply. One of the minerals is iodine, essential to thyroid health.

If you suspect that you might have an underactive thyroid gland, read chapter 4 on thyroid health and take the thyroid health quiz. Addressing this issue is very important, not only for your weight loss program to be effective, but for your heart health as well.

In the end, heart disease may result from any number of causes. What contributes to heart disease in one individual may not affect another person. It is so important to look at all the factors and make the necessary changes in your lifestyle.

FATS FOR LIFE!

For centuries saturated fats have been a healthy part of traditional diets—healthy fats from free-range, grass-fed animals and oils such as coconut oil, which are heavily saturated.

On the other hand, expeller-pressed and solvent-extracted seed-based oils have been around for less than 100 years. These polyunsaturated oils are very susceptible to rancidity (oxidation) and easily turn to trans-fatty acids when hydrogenated and oxidize when heated to high temperatures. They must be heavily refined and then hydrogenated to become a solid fat like margarine, which is loaded with toxic trans-fatty acids. Many studies now show that these oils lead to modern diseases and sicknesses that were not common among people eating traditional diets.

The much-maligned saturated fats—which many Americans have tried so hard to avoid—do not appear to be the major cause of heart disease or obesity. They have been a part of healthy traditional diets for centuries and have not been implicated in weight gain. Coconut oil, in particular, has been particularly helpful for weight loss and beneficial for people who suffer with hypothyroid, diabetes, chronic fatigue syndrome, irritable bowel syndrome (IBS), Crohn's disease, and other digestive disorders.

The Coconut Diet takes these healthful fats from the coconut, and helps you learn how to add them to your favorite foods and dishes in order to reap the benefits of weight loss and improved health. This delicious fat makes everything taste great and almost seems too good to be a weight loss–promoting ingredient. Add to that a host of health benefits and you just might be calling it your "miracle oil."

Chapter 4

Thyroid Health: A Weight Loss Advantage

About 13 million people suffer from low thyroid. This is a primary reason why some people can't lose weight on a low-carb diet, or any diet, for that matter. If you have hypothyroidism or suspect that you do, this chapter may be key in helping you lose the weight you want. If you think you might have a sluggish thyroid but aren't sure, you could take the Thyroid Health Quiz on page 78. If you know you don't have low thyroid, you can skip this chapter. And if you don't have trouble losing weight, the next chapter might not apply as well. You may be ready to start The Coconut Diet in part II.

Research points to the fact that an underactive thyroid gland might be the number one cause of weight problems, especially among women. Because thyroid hormones are required for normal health and activity of every cell in the body, it just makes sense that a lack of these hormones will have a detrimental effect on organs and tissues. If thyroid function is not corrected, ideal weight may never be achieved.

The thyroid gland is the body's metabolic thermostat, controlling body temperature, energy use, and growth rate in children. The thyroid produces thyroid hormones, which control the health of organs and the speed at which the body metabolizes food. Simply put, it affects the operation of all our body's cells, tissues, and organs.

Many people experience a number of symptoms when they have a sluggish thyroid: fatigue, depression, weight gain, cold hands and feet, low body temperature, sensitivity to cold, a feeling of always being chilled, joint pain, headaches, menstrual disorders, insomnia, dry skin, puffy eyes, hair loss, brittle nails, constipation, mental dullness, frequent infections, hoarse voice, ringing in the ears, dizziness, and low sex drive.

People that are hypothyroid are also more likely to experience related conditions such as high cholesterol, carpal tunnel syndrome, chronic fatigue syndrome, fibromyalgia, difficult menopause, mitral valve prolapse, and fibrocystic breasts.

An underactive thyroid can lead to hormonal imbalance, which is often a factor in premenstrual syndrome (PMS). A number of experts believe that PMS is due to an imbalance of hormones, namely an excess of estrogen and a deficiency of progesterone. Studies have revealed that a large percentage of women suffering from PMS (symptoms such as moodiness, irritability, bloating, fatigue, and craving for sweets at least one week before menstruation) have shown evidence of poor thyroid function.

Because many of these symptoms are general and nonspecific or seemingly unrelated, many health care professionals do not think about sluggish thyroid as a potential cause, and the condition goes undiagnosed and untreated.

DETERMINING LOW THYROID

If some of the symptoms just mentioned ring true for you, but you are not sure if you have low thyroid, take the Thyroid Health Quiz on page 78.

I also recommend that you take your body temperature for four mornings in a row before you get out of bed. Shake down a glass thermometer to below 95 degrees Fahrenheit and place it by your bed before you go to sleep. Upon waking, place the thermometer in your armpit for a full 10 minutes. It is important to move as little as possible during this time. Remain still with your eyes closed. Don't get up for any reason. After 10 minutes, record the temperature and date. This should be done for four consecutive mornings.

Individuals with normal functioning thyroids have a resting basal body temperature between 97.6 and 98.2. Basal body temperatures below this range may reflect hypothyroidism or an underactive thyroid.

HYPOTHYROIDISM REACHING
EPIDEMIC PROPORTIONS

In 1995, researchers studied 25,862 participants at the Colorado statewide health fair. They discovered that among people not taking thyroid medication, 8.9 percent were hypothyroid (underactive thyroid) and 1.1 percent were hyperthyroid (overactive thyroid). This indicates 9.9 percent of the population had a thyroid problem that had most likely gone unrecognized. These figures suggest that nationally, there may be as many as 13 million Americans with an undiagnosed thyroid problem.[1]

In his book *What Your Doctor May Not Tell You About Hypothyroidism*, the endocrinologist Kenneth Blanchard, M.D., says that doctors are always told that TSH (thyroid stimulating hormone) measurement is the test that gives a definitive answer about the health of the thyroid. He thinks that's fundamentally wrong. The pituitary TSH is controlled not just by how much T4 and T3 is in circulation, but how T4 gets converted to T3. Excess T3 generated at the pituitary level can falsely suppress TSH. Hence, many people who are simply tested for TSH levels and are found to be within "normal" range are, in fact, suffering from thyroid problems that are going undetected.[2]

Ridha Arem, M.D., associate professor of medicine in the Division of Endocrinology and Metabolism at Baylor College of Medicine, agrees. He says that hypothyroidism may exist despite "normal range" TSH levels. In his book, *The Thyroid Solution*, he says:

Many people may be suffering from minute imbalances that have not yet resulted in abnormal blood tests. If we included people with low-grade hypothyroidism whose blood tests are normal, the frequency of hypothyroidism would no doubt exceed 10 percent of the population. What is of special concern, though, is that many people whose test results are dismissed as normal could continue to have symptoms of an underactive thyroid. Their moods, emotions, and overall well-being are affected by this imbalance, yet they are not receiving the care they need to get to the root of their problems. Even if the TSH level is in the lower segment of normal range, a person may still be suffering from low-grade hypothyroidism. Thus, if we were to include those who may be suffering from "low-grade hypothyroidism" the number could well be double the 13 million estimate.[3]

THYROID CANCER

The statistics on thyroid cancer in the United States also tell a disturbing tale. Since 1990, cancer statistics show that the overall thyroid cancer incidence across all ages and races in the United States has been subject to a statistically significant annual increase of 1.4. That increase was highest among females (1.6 percent per annum). Also worth noting is that between 1975 and 1996 the incidence of thyroid cancer has risen 42.1 percent in the United States. This increase was particularly notable in women and most recent figures (1996) show that the incidence of thyroid cancer has climbed to 8.0 per 100,000. The National Cancer Institute (NCI) notes that "the preponderance of thyroid cancer in females suggest that hormonal factors may mediate disease occurrence.[4]"

Especially alarming is the rate of thyroid cancer among children. The NCI (National Cancer Institute) has reported that the most prevalent carcinomas in American children and adolescents younger than 20 years was thyroid carcinoma at 35.5 percent—more prevalent than the highly publicized melanomas (30.9 percent). Approximately 75 percent of the thyroid carcinomas occurred in adolescents 15 to 19 years of age.[5]

WHAT IS CAUSING THIS EPIDEMIC?

Though more research is needed, it is generally accepted that diet plays a major role in thyroid health. For decades most people have known that low iodine intake leads to low thyroid function and eventually to goiter. Iodized salt was intended to solve this problem, but it has not been our salvation. Refined table salt (sodium chloride) does not seem to be a good delivery system.

Add to that the number of foods frequently eaten in this culture that are known as *goitrogens* (iodine blockers) and a picture develops as to why thyroid problems are on the rise. Two goitrogens are quite prevalent in the American diet—peanuts (and peanut butter) and soybeans (which include soy oil found in many commercially made salad dressings and packaged foods) and textured vegetable protein, which is used most often in prepared foods such as veggie burgers, energy bars, and fillers in commercially made snacks and baked goods.

Add to that the rise of industrialization, corporate farming, iodine-deficient soil, and mass production of food, all negatively changing the modern-day food supply. Many studies also show detrimental effects of refined sugars and grains on thyroid health. These foods are very taxing on the thyroid gland, and Americans consume them in large quantities.

Environmental stress such as chemical pollutants, pesticides, mercury, and fluoride are also tough on the thyroid. A growing body of evidence suggests that fluoride, which is prevalent in toothpaste and water treatment, may inhibit the functioning of the thyroid gland. Additionally, mercury may diminish thyroid function because it displaces the trace mineral selenium, and selenium is involved in conversion of thyroid hormones T4 to T3.

THE FATS AND OILS CONNECTION

Many oils can negatively affect thyroid health. Many Americans prepare their food or eat restaurant food made with a variety of polyunsaturated oils. These oils are also plentiful in commercially manufactured foods that line grocery store shelves.

Expeller-pressed or solvent-extracted oils became a major part of the American diet only in the past century. It is possible they are among the worst offenders of thyroid health. These oils are known as vegetable or seed oils and most of them are polyunsaturated. The most common source of these oils used in commercially prepared foods is soybeans. A careful examination of food labels reveals how often this oil is used. (Often labels simply state "vegetable oil.")

Large-scale cultivation of soybeans in the United States began after World War II and quickly increased to 140 billion pounds per year. Most of the crops are produced for animal feed and soy oil for hydrogenated fats such as margarine and shortening. Today, it is nearly impossible to eat at restaurants or buy packaged foods that don't have soy oil in the ingredients.

Ray Peat, Ph.D., a physiologist who has worked with progesterone and related hormones since 1968, says that the sudden surge of polyunsaturated oils into the food chain post–World War II has caused many changes in hormones. He writes:

> Their [polyunsaturated oils] best understood effect is their interference with the function of the thyroid gland. Unsaturated oils block thyroid hormone secretion, its movement in the circulatory system, and the response of tissues to the hormone. When the thyroid hormone is deficient, the body is generally exposed to increased levels of estrogen. The thyroid hormone is essential for making the "protective hormones" progesterone and pregnenolone, so these hormones are lowered when anything interferes with the function of the thyroid. The thyroid hormone is required for using and eliminating cholesterol, so cholesterol is likely to be raised by anything which blocks the thyroid function.[6]

A growing body of research alludes to soy's detrimental effects on the thyroid gland. Now that researchers know that soybeans are goitrogens, which block iodine, much of their work currently centers on the *phytoestrogens* (phyto means plant) that are found in soy. In the

I didn't realize how much hypothyroidism was affecting my life until I started on virgin coconut oil and suddenly had energy like the Energizer Bunny! I gave up the "white toxins" (wheat flour, refined sugar, potatoes, and other high-glycemic index foods). I combined this diet with coconut oil and it has made a tremendous difference in my hormonal balance, mood stability, stamina, and overall energy. I'm slowly but steadily losing a little bit of weight. I feel *great*!

—*Julia*

1960s, when soy was introduced into infant formulas, it was shown that soy was goitrogenic and caused goiters in babies. When iodine was supplemented, the incidence of goiter reduced dramatically.

A retrospective epidemiological study showed that teenaged children with a diagnosis of autoimmune thyroid disease were significantly more likely to have received soy formula as infants (18 of 59 children—31 percent) when compared with healthy siblings (9 of 76—12 percent) or control group children (7 of 54—13 percent).[7]

When healthy individuals without any previous thyroid disease were fed 30 grams of pickled soybeans per day for one month, researchers reported goiter and elevated individual thyroid stimulating hormone (TSH) levels (although still within the normal range) in 37 healthy iodine-sufficient adults. One month after stopping soybean consumption, individual TSH values decreased to the original levels and goiters were reduced in size.[8]

COCONUT OIL: A HEALTHY CHOICE FOR YOUR THYROID

Traditionally, polyunsaturated oils such as soy oil have been used for livestock feed because they cause the animals to gain weight.[9] These oils are made up of long-chain fatty acids (LCTs)—the kind

I am just now jumping on the coconut oil bandwagon (about three weeks now) and I'm really starting to feel *great*. I have suffered from severe migraines for the past 25 years, the last 15 becoming increasingly severe, coinciding with the addition of soy and the "low-fat mentality" to my diet. Nothing helped! I should be experiencing my premenstrual migraine by now and instead I feel like I could climb Mount Everest! Also I wondered if it decreased the waist-to-hip ratio because mine has gone from 7.2 (all my life) to 7. I think I had a sluggish thyroid, with a low body temperature of between 96 and 96.8 [degrees Fahrenheit]. Now it's starting to climb for the first time in years.

—*V. Potter*

I have had a problem with a sluggish metabolism and weight gain since having children. Even a no-calorie diet (fast) for five days did not work. As soon as I started taking virgin coconut oil the fat began to melt and I have lost 20 pounds. Over the same period, my 13-year-old daughter, who was very chubby and very worried about it, but could not [find] the self-control to renounce some of her favorite fatty foods, lost about 10 pounds. She now has the perfect figure, to her great joy! Pants she was bulging out of a year ago hang loose on her!

—*Sharon*

of fatty acids that promote weight gain. Conversely, coconut oil—made up primarily of medium-chain fatty acids—has caused animals to lose weight. This was discovered in the 1940s when farmers tried using coconut oil to fatten their animals and discovered that it made them lean and active instead. Medium-chain fatty acids (MCTs) are known to increase metabolism and promote weight loss. An increased metabolic rate is key to healthy weight management. This is good news for people who suffer with low thyroid function. There have been scores of testimonies to this effect.

OILS AND OXIDATIVE STRESS

One of the reasons the long-chain triglycerides (LCTs) in vegetable oils are so damaging to the thyroid is that they oxidize quickly and become rancid. To prevent rancidity, food manufacturers highly refine vegetable oils. Considerable research has shown that trans-fatty acids, present when vegetable oils are highly refined, are especially damaging to cell tissue and can have a negative effect on the thyroid gland as well as on health in general.

Because the longer-chain fatty acids are deposited in cells more often as rancid, oxidized fat, the body's ability to convert the thyroid hormone T4 to T3 (which creates the enzymes needed to convert fats to energy) is impaired. When this breakdown occurs, one can develop symptoms typical of hypothyroidism.

Dr. Ray Peat says:

> When the oils are stored in our tissues, they are much warmer, and more directly exposed to oxygen than they would be in the seeds, and so their tendency to oxidize is very great. These oxidative processes can damage enzymes and other parts of cells, and especially their ability to produce energy. The enzymes which break down proteins are inhibited by unsaturated fats; these enzymes are needed not only for digestion, but also for production of thyroid hormones, clot removal, immunity, and the general adaptability of cells. The risks of abnormal blood clotting, inflammation, immune deficiency, shock, aging, obesity, and cancer are increased. Thyroid [hormones] and progesterone are decreased.
>
> Since the unsaturated oils block protein digestion in the stomach, we can be malnourished even while "eating well." There are many changes in hormones caused by unsaturated fats. Their best understood effect is their interference with the function of the thyroid gland. Unsaturated oils block thyroid hormone secretion, its movement in the circulatory system, and the response of tissues to the hormone. Coconut oil is unique in its ability to prevent weight gain or cure obesity, by

I have had rheumatoid arthritis for 23 years and have found a big correlation among general hormone balance, adrenal function, and symptoms. Since I have been using therapeutic amounts of coconut oil, my hormones, including adrenal hormones, have been in much better balance. And my thyroid is back in balance, too. I have lost 27 pounds through improving my thyroid with virgin coconut oil and cutting out refined carbs. My energy (something you don't have if your adrenals are shot) is amazing now.

—Julia

I have experienced [thyroid] problems . . . body temperature not going above 97 degrees, cold hands and feet, can't lose weight, fatigued, slow heart rate, can't sleep some nights, dry skin, etc. . . . My doctor did the [thyroid] test and it came back normal. I am 46 and perimenopausal. My naturopath symptomatically diagnosed me with hypothyroidism. She explained the blood tests currently used by allopathic medicine are not sensitive enough. I started on the [coconut] oil five weeks ago.

In the first week I noticed my body temperature had risen and my resting heart rate had gone from 49 to 88 beats per minute. This has since settled to 66. My energy is now really high and I am slowly losing the weight—three pounds in the past five weeks. I also had been taking flaxseed oil and gamma linoleic acid oil but have stopped eating every other oil but what Dr. Raymond Peat recommends, which is coconut oil, olive oil and butter (obviously using the last two very sparingly). I take three tablespoons of coconut oil daily. I have discussed this with my naturopath and have given her all the written material on it. She's very open to knowing more about it.

—Cindy

stimulating metabolism. It is quickly metabolized, and functions in some ways as an antioxidant.[10]

Because coconut oil is saturated and very stable (unrefined coconut oil has a shelf life of about two years at room temperature), the body is not burdened with oxidative stress as it is with the vegetable oils. Unlike vegetable oils, coconut oil does not require the enzyme stress that prevents T4 to T3 hormone conversion, because it is processed differently in the body and does not need to be broken down by enzyme-dependent processes.

Since the liver is the main organ where damage occurs from oxidized and rancid oils that cause cell membrane damage, and where much of the conversion of T4 to T3 takes place, replacing long-chain fatty acids with medium-chain fatty acids found in coconut oil can, in time, help rebuild cell membranes and increases enzyme production that will help in promoting the conversion of T4 to T3 hormones.

More research in this area may be necessary, but in the meantime, those switching from polyunsaturated oils to coconut oil are reporting many positive results.

CORRECTING THYROID PROBLEMS

Rather than simply taking thyroid medication, it is very important to identify the underlying causes of low thyroid function. You may need to take medication until you have corrected the underlying problem, but simply taking thyroid hormone replacement drugs for a lifetime does not feed the thyroid or correct the problem.

David Frahm, N.D., says, "Instead of feeding the thyroid and bringing it back into full function in the body, they're [medications] simply by-passing it."[11] This does help increase energy to some degree when the body is supplied with some of the hormones it is supposed to make on its own, but none of these drugs actually restore thyroid function.

I have been taking virgin coconut oil for about two to three months. Before then, my thyroid results were borderline low. After two months of one tablespoon a day [of coconut oil], they are now mid-normal range. They have never been this high. I do *not* take any thyroid [medication]. Also my cholesterol is still the same as well as my LDL, but my HDL [the good cholesterol] rose 10 whole points from 43 to 53! This is a miracle for me.

—*Lori*

Since the thyroid makes a hormone called calcitonin that allows for absorption of calcium, people who take just thyroid hormone replacement drugs won't fix the underlying problem and calcium absorption will remain impaired. Often these people will experience bone loss, and this is the best explanation as to why many people with hypothyroidism also experience osteoporosis.

Before discontinuing thyroid hormone replacement medication, always check with your doctor. In the meantime, there are a number of things you can do to feed your thyroid gland and improve its health.

As you incorporate thyroid-supporting solutions into your daily routine, watch for signals that your thyroid is beginning to improve, such as rapid heartbeat and a rise in body temperature. Many complementary and alternative health doctors address such symptoms as a "healing crisis." At this point, if taking thyroid medication, it would be wise to consult your physician for retesting.

WHAT YOU CAN DO TO NOURISH YOUR THYROID

A number of nutrients and foods have been shown to contribute to healthy thyroid function. As you incorporate these into your diet, you should notice an improvement in your thyroid health. If your attempts at weight loss have been discouraging, you should notice that weight management greatly improves. Here's what you can do.

Eat Only Healthy Fats and Oils

A number of health professionals now recommend that we eat only virgin coconut oil, extra virgin olive oil, and butter; it is best to eat butter sparingly. Coconut oil can be used in place of butter for many dishes. Coconut oil is one of the most stable oils available because of its medium-chain triglycerides. Avoid all other cooking oils. Never eat margarine. And read every label on packaged foods. If vegetable oil or soybean oil is listed, don't buy it. Be aware that most commercial salad dressings and mayonnaise contain soybean oil or another polyunsaturated oil.

You could benefit from preparing your own salad dressings and mayonnaise. You can take mayo-free salad dressings along when you travel or eat out. If that is not possible, ask for lemon slices or vinegar and olive oil and prepare your own dressing on the spot. Restaurant-fried foods are particularly worrisome because the oils used are heated to very high temperatures for a variety of dishes and often used over and over for deep frying; they are loaded with trans-fatty acids. Whenever you can, prepare your own healthy food at home, where you can control the ingredients.

Many people who have improved their thyroid health have lost weight and increased their energy by including two to three tablespoons of virgin coconut oil in their diet each day. There are a number of ways to accomplish this. Cooking with coconut oil is the most obvious method. It tastes great with every food from sautéed onions or vegetables to eggs and baked goods.

You may also want to add one or two extra tablespoons of coconut oil to your diet daily. Smoothies are one way to accomplish this. You could try the Low-Carb Coconut Smoothie (page 153). I also developed 101 smoothie recipes available in *The Ultimate Smoothie Book* and you can add coconut oil to any of them, or try the Coconut Treats recipe (page 211).

I make moussaka using coconut oil instead of olive oil. The first time I tried it, I was "freaking out" as the exotic island coconut aroma wafted through the house while I was working on [this] Mediterranean recipe. I'm Greek and this is a classic Greek recipe. Who has ever heard of using coconut [oil] to make moussaka, but I will tell you it works! It works just great. And my guests could not tell the difference.

—*Marie*

Consume Plenty of Iodine-Rich Foods

Iodine is most abundant in sea vegetables, cranberries, fish, and eggs. You can find a variety of dried sea vegetables at most health food stores, Asian markets, and some grocery stores. Add a strip of kombu to soups or bean dishes; sprinkle black seaweed on salads or add to soup. Season foods with dulse or kelp powder in place of salt. Use Celtic sea salt (also called gray salt) whenever possible—it is loaded with minerals including iodine. Eat more fish, especially the smaller coldwater fish such as salmon (avoid farm raised), mackerel, halibut, sole, sardines, and snapper. Avoid the larger fish such as tuna and swordfish; they tend to be higher in mercury, which interferes with thyroid function. Choose cage-free, hormone- and antibiotic-free eggs; they're healthier and they offer a good source of iodine.

Take Vitamin and Mineral Supplements

In addition to iodine, a number of nutrients have been shown to contribute to thyroid health; they include zinc, selenium, manganese, chromium, B vitamins, vitamin C, vitamin E, and vitamin A.

The thyroid gland requires very high levels of vitamin A. Individuals with hypothyroidism have an impaired ability to convert beta-carotene to vitamin A, so care should be taken to include supplementation of vitamin A in addition to beta-carotene. Cod liver oil is a very good source of natural vitamin A. (Choose cod liver oil from cod caught in Icelandic or Norwegian waters, where fish are less likely to have high mercury levels.)

Kelp tablets have been used for many years as a natural treatment for sluggish thyroid since kelp is an excellent source of iodine. Kelp can support thyroid and pituitary health. Look for kelp tablets with a source from Icelandic or Norwegian waters. Also, iodine drops may be helpful. (See Resources.)

Selenium is involved in conversion of T4 to T3 hormones and low selenium levels could lead to low T3 levels. Be sure to include foods that are high in selenium, such as raw Brazil nuts, red Swiss chard, garlic, lamb, eggs, mushrooms, and chicken. You may also need to take supplemental selenium.

Because mercury will displace selenium, consider a *heavy metal detoxification* program, especially if you have had mercury amalgam fillings, have eaten a lot of tuna, or have been exposed to mercury in any other manner.

The mineral chromium helps metabolize carbohydrates and fat. It is also important for hormonal activity, especially of insulin, and plays a role in thyroid hormone metabolism.

The amino acid L-tyrosine may be beneficial as well. L-tyrosine and iodine are important nutrients that work together in the production of thyroid hormones.

Juicing Can Be Restorative

Vegetable juicing can be particularly helpful in restoring health to the thyroid as well as the entire body. A steady diet of radishes (yes, you can juice them) and radish juice can be quite beneficial. A sulfur compound found in the radish is a regulator of thyroxine and calcitonin (a peptide hormone). When enough of this sulfur compound is circulating in the bloodstream, the thyroid is less apt to over- or underproduce these hormones. Try a thyroid tonic that includes the juice of carrots, cucumber, celery, radishes, and lemon. To that you can add a dash of powdered kelp or dulse for a boost of iodine.

Cranberry is another helpful juice. Because the bogs of Massachusetts where cranberries are grown are near the sea, cranberries contain iodine.[12] You can juice cranberries with a low-sugar apple such as pippin or Granny Smith and add a squeeze of lemon for an absolutely delicious cranberry juice cocktail and, unlike the store-bought cranberry juice (except for unsweetened cranberry concentrate), it will not have added sugar. For other juice recipes, see *The Juice Lady's Guide to Juicing for Health* (Avery, 1999).

LIFESTYLE MODIFICATIONS

As you nourish your thyroid, you also want to avoid the foods and substances that can tax this important gland or interfere with nutrient absorption. Following are a few suggestions that can make an important difference in assisting thyroid function.

Avoid Goitrogens

Excessive ingestion of certain foods known as goitrogens can block iodine from being absorbed by the thyroid gland; these include turnips, cabbage, mustard, cassava root, pine nuts, millet, peanuts, and soybeans. Until your thyroid health is restored, you may want to avoid these foods completely or eat them sparingly. When your thyroid gland is healthy again and you no longer have symptoms, you could include them occasionally, but you probably should never eat them daily.

Watch out for such foods as soybean oil, often found in commercial salad dressings; mayonnaise; textured vegetable protein, often used as a filler and found in many vegetarian packaged foods; and peanuts, peanut oil, and peanut butter. These products are included in many commercially packaged foods, snacks, and treats. It is interesting to note that in Asian cultures soy is eaten only in small quantities and in traditional forms that have been fermented.

Omit All Substances That Tax the Thyroid

Foods that are the most taxing on the thyroid are foods many Americans consume every day, such as refined grains, sugar and sweets, caffeine (coffee, black tea, green tea, sodas, and chocolate), refined, hydrogenated and partially hydrogenated oils, and alcohol.

Avoid all refined grains, such as white and wheat bread, rolls, biscuits, pancakes, pizza dough, pasta, and buns. One of America's favorites—the peanut butter sandwich—is a perfect example of a really bad choice for the thyroid. It combines refined grain bread (a taxing food for the thyroid) and peanut butter (a goitrogen). Avoid sugar in all forms, such as white sugar, corn syrup, maple syrup, honey, molasses, fructose, and brown rice syrup, and avoid all desserts.

Use stevia, an herbal sweetener that can be found at most health food stores. Or try birch sugar (xylitol) or Lo Han Guo.

In addition, emotional stress such as anger, grief, guilt, anxiety, and fear can be very taxing on the thyroid. You may benefit from interpersonal work dealing with, and letting go of, negative emotions. Also, giving birth, environmental stress such as industrial pollutants, pesticides (a clear case for buying organic foods!), metal toxicity, *Candida albicans* (yeast overgrowth), and medical stress (radiation, X-rays, and drugs) all strain the thyroid gland.

Limit Exposure to Fluoride and Mercury

It is beneficial to avoid fluoride and mercury as much as possible. To that end, a water filtration/purification system that removes fluoride and other chemicals is worth the purchase. Buy fluoride-free tooth-paste from a health food store. Have mercury amalgam fillings removed from your mouth by a dentist trained to remove them properly so as not to further poison your system. And consume smaller coldwater fish such as salmon, mackerel, sole, sardines, and halibut that usually have less mercury.

Cleansing Protocols

Many people have benefited greatly from various cleansing programs such as colon cleansing, the liver cleanse, gallbladder cleanse, kidney cleanse (all in Phase II), and a *Candida albicans* cleanse. The 7-Day Liver Cleanse may be particularly helpful because a well-functioning liver can greatly assist your thyroid; some of the T4 hormones are converted to T3 in the liver. A congested liver will not perform such functions efficiently. (See chapter 7, "Phase II: Cleansing—A Weight Loss Advantage.")

Exercise

Exercise is particularly important in helping to correct low thyroid function. Exercise stimulates thyroid gland secretion and increases tissue sensitivity to thyroid hormones. Choose exercises that fit your energy level. You may start by walking and perhaps taking a stretch class. Weight-bearing exercise is particularly important to prevent osteoporosis. Work up to exercises such as step aerobics or fast walking that increase your heart rate—and are excellent for the cardiovascular system. Studies prove that exercise increases metabolic rate, an important aspect in weight loss. Jumping on a rebounder (mini-trampoline) is very beneficial for the organs and lymphatic system. Also, a machine called the "lymphasizer" (also known as a chi machine or swing machine) can be very beneficial to move the lymph (see Resources). Whatever you do, get up and move. Your energy will improve as you do more exercising, even if you begin with only 15 minutes a day.

HOW LONG WILL IT TAKE TO RESTORE THYROID HEALTH?

The beneficial effects of a comprehensive treatment of low thyroid are usually evident within two to three weeks after starting therapy. However, it is important to emphasize that while symptoms may be alleviated and people with hypothyroidism may experience a greater sense of well-being, in most cases, treatment for this condition requires a lifelong commitment. It's worth it. You can look forward to a life of vibrant health, weight maintenance, and lowered risks of degenerative disease.

TYING IT ALL TOGETHER

The best approach to maintaining a healthy thyroid and proper weight management is to follow the advice in this chapter. By eating healthy foods that will nourish and not damage the thyroid, adding the nutrients recommended, avoiding the foods and substances that tax the thyroid, and cleansing the body, you can expect to see improvement in thyroid function in just a few weeks.[13]

Important dietary changes include replacing soy oil and other polyunsaturated oils with healthy oils, the best being coconut oil, and getting sufficient iodine to feed the thyroid gland.

If you need to lose weight, the pounds should melt away naturally as you follow these suggestions. And, you can look forward to living a higher quality of life.

THYROID HEALTH QUIZ
(SYMPTOMS OF AN UNDERACTIVE THYROID)

Score 1 point for each symptom that applies to you.

_____	Appetite problems—severely reduced or excessive
_____	Bloating or indigestion after eating
_____	Low body temperature (below 97.6—resting)
_____	Weight gain
_____	Mucus accumulation
_____	Hoarse throat
_____	Cold hands and feet
_____	Puffy eyes
_____	Constipation
_____	Decreased sweating
_____	Dry mouth—drinking water doesn't help much
_____	Intolerance to cold or heat
_____	Poor digestion of animal products
_____	Poor absorption of minerals
_____	Sluggish lymph drainage
_____	Swelling—ankles, eyelids, face, feet, hands, lymph nodes, throat
_____	Spleen or liver problems
_____	Calcium deficiency
_____	Carpal tunnel syndrome
_____	Left arm weakness
_____	Muscle/joint problems—knees, elbows, etc.
_____	Numbness in fingers
_____	Stiff neck
_____	Tenderness in lower ribs
_____	Brittle nails
_____	Grooves or ridges in nails
_____	Thin, peeling nails
_____	Slow-growing nails
_____	White spots on nails (this can also be a zinc deficiency)
_____	Fluttering in ears

_____	Occasional stinging in eyes
_____	Poor vision
_____	Impotency
_____	Loss of libido/low sex drive
_____	Miscarriages
_____	Premature deliveries
_____	Spontaneous abortions
_____	Stillbirths
_____	Coarse, dry hair
_____	Hair loss
_____	Loss of hair on arms, underarms, legs, eyebrows, scalp
_____	Elevated cholesterol
_____	Enlargement of heart
_____	Heart pain
_____	Hypertension
_____	Pain in diaphragm
_____	Heart palpitations
_____	Impaired heart function
_____	Slower heart rate
_____	Sense of pressure (compression) on chest
_____	PMS
_____	Prolonged or heavy menstrual bleeding
_____	Light menstrual flow
_____	Shorter menstrual cycle
_____	Bi-polarity (manic-depression)
_____	Depression
_____	Difficulty concentrating
_____	Emotionally unstable
_____	Fatigue/lack of energy
_____	Forgetfulness
_____	Inability to "drag oneself from bed"
_____	Lethargy
_____	Nervousness
_____	Restlessness
_____	Shyness

Continued

_____ Tendency to cry easily
_____ Chronic mucus in head/nose (thyroid governs mucus
           production)
_____ Shortness of breath
_____ Difficulty drawing deep breath
_____ Gasping for air occasionally
_____ Intolerance to closed, stuffy rooms
_____ Loss of smell
_____ Need for fresh air
_____ Sleep disturbances
_____ Grinding teeth during sleep
_____ Loss of hearing

A score of 20 points or more may be indicative of an underactive thyroid. Although the thyroid quiz can help you determine your thyroid health, ultimately the best method for diagnosis is clinical evaluation by a physician knowledgeable in thyroid health. See a physician who can treat your condition holistically.

Chapter 5

Special Help When Diets Don't Work

If you have tried in vain to lose weight, take heart. Everybody is unique. There is no one-size-fits-all approach to weight loss or nutrition. This chapter explores some of the reasons why people don't lose weight on various diets, including low-carb plans, and tells why The Coconut Diet can help when combined with some of the suggestions herein. This chapter offers various steps to overcome certain health issues that may have been preventing you from losing those extra pounds and tips to overcome emotional or binge eating.

WHY SOME PEOPLE CAN'T LOSE WEIGHT

Though low-carb diets work for many people, individuals who suffer with certain health or emotional responses that involve food find it very difficult to lose weight. A healthy low-carb diet is important to follow. However, unless the physical disorder or the emotional eating is addressed, some individuals may spend a lifetime trying unsuccessfully to lose weight. The Coconut Diet can change all that along with the special help in this chapter.

Perhaps the doctors have given up on you. Maybe someone has told you there's no hope that you'll lose weight and that you may as well learn to live with it. Don't believe it! Very often when problems that cause both ill health and weight gain are corrected, the weight melts off naturally. When all the systems of the body come into harmony, when you experience biochemical and hormonal balance, when you detoxify your organs of elimination, and correct root causes of ill health, you can achieve and maintain a healthy weight.

The late Dr. Robert C. Atkins said that about 20 percent of the people on the Atkins diet don't lose weight because of yeasts known as *Candida albicans*.[1] Candidiasis is one of the conditions that is covered in this chapter, along with chronic fatigue syndrome, fibromyalgia (hypothyroid is covered in chapter 4), digestive disorders such as irritable bowl syndrome, leaky gut syndrome, Crohn's disease, and colitis, plus a section on emotional and binge eating.

Cleansing the body is one of the most important steps you can take to correct any of these conditions. When everything in your body is free-flowing, and you eliminate toxins and wastes quickly and easily, and when you feed your body an abundance of nutrients, the body's natural processes begin healing many ailments and the weight starts melting away. Remove everything that hinders the body's healing process, such as toxins, waste, and poor food choices, and provide the body with the materials it needs to do its innate work of restoration and balance, and the body will heal itself.

If you suffer from any of the conditions discussed here, begin with Phase II of The Coconut Diet and follow the food guidelines in Phase I. Or, if you have already completed Phase I, you may include the food choices in Phase III (unless not advised for your condition), while incorporating the specific recommendations in this chapter that apply to your needs.

CANDIDIASIS

Candida albicans are usually benign yeasts (or fungus) that naturally inhabit the folds and creases of the digestive tract and in women also in the vaginal tract. They normally live in harmonious relationship with beneficial intestinal flora, also known as *probiotics*. In healthy people, *C. albicans* does not present a problem because the good bacteria that also inhabit the gut keep the yeasts in check.

These good bacteria can be easily destroyed by the use of anti-biotics and other medications, allowing *C. albicans* to flourish. Other factors mostly connected with the twenty-first-century lifestyle, such as diets rich in sugars, refined carbohydrates, alcohol, birth control pills, pregnancy, hormonal changes, and stress, encourage yeasts to grow out of control.[2]

Thought to affect more than 40 million Americans, *C. albicans* is now being recognized as a complex medical syndrome known as *chronic candidiasis* or *yeast syndrome*.[3] These organisms attach themselves to the intestinal wall where they compete with cells for nutrients, thus creating nutrient deficiencies. This overgrowth of yeast is believed to cause widespread symptoms in virtually every system of the body, with the gastrointestinal, genitourinary, endocrine, nervous, and immune systems being the most susceptible.[4]

This syndrome can cause a host of uncomfortable symptoms such as fatigue, vaginitis, weight gain, immune system dysfunction, depression, digestive disorders, ear and sinus irritation or infection, intense itching, chemical sensitivities, canker sores, and ringworm. Some patients say they feel "sick all over." If you think you may have a yeast overgrowth, I recommend you fill in the Candida Questionnaire found on page 101.

Predisposing Factors

Chronic candidiasis has many predisposing factors, such as altered bowel flora, decreased digestive secretions, dietary factors such as consuming too much sugar and too many other high-carbohydrate foods, drugs (particularly antibiotics), immune dysfunction, impaired liver function, nutrient deficiencies, and underlying disease states. Simply going after the yeasts and killing them off, whether using natural or synthetic antifungal agents, will not get to the root of what caused candidiasis in the first place. It's a lot like cutting leaves off a weed. It is vitally important to address all the factors that predisposed the yeast overgrowth and get to the root of the problem.

Correcting the Problem

In addition to using antifungal agents, it's very important to address the predisposing factors. Here's what I recommend.

Follow a Candida-control diet. The Coconut Diet is especially suited for *C. albicans* sufferers since the early phases of the diet eliminate grains, fruit, alcohol, sugars, and other carbs that quickly turn to sugar, which *C. albicans* is known to feed on. In addition, eliminate all natural sugars when cleansing the body of yeasts, because sugars are the primary food for yeasts. Omit all milk and dairy products as well, because milk lactose promotes overgrowth of yeasts. Also, avoid all mold- and yeast-containing foods such as alcohol, cheese, dried fruit, bread, and peanuts. Eliminate food allergens. Candidiasis sufferers may need to avoid these foods even after completing Phase I of the program, as *C. albicans* infections are known to be opportunistic and very difficult to overcome if the condition is systemic (the yeast has spread to other areas outside the intestines to other parts of the body). It is best to stick with this diet until you are symptom-free and yeast-free.

Include plenty of coconut oil in your diet. Research shows that the medium chain fatty acids in coconut oil kill *C. albicans.* Caprylic acid is one fatty acid found in coconut oil that has been used for quite some time in fighting *C. albicans* infections. William Crook, M.D., the author of *The Yeast Connection* and developer of the Candida Questionnaire, reports that many physicians have used caprylic acid successfully for yeast overgrowth and that it works especially well for those patients who have adverse reactions to antifungal drugs. Besides caprylic acid, two other medium-chain fatty acids (lauric and capric acid) found in coconut oil have been shown to kill *C. albicans.* A study done at the University of Iceland showed "capric acid, a 10-carbon saturated fatty acid, causes the fastest and most effective killing of all three strains of *Candida albicans* tested, leaving the cytoplasm disorganized and shrunken because of a disrupted or disintegrated plasma membrane. Lauric acid, a 12-carbon saturated fatty acid, was the most active at lower concentrations and after a longer incubation time."[5] This study makes the case that all the medium chain fatty acids in coconut oil work together to kill *C. albicans.*

Interestingly, people who eat a lot of coconuts live in areas where yeast and fungi are extremely plentiful, yet they are rarely troubled by yeast infections. Women in the Philippines, who eat their traditional coconut-based diet, rarely, if ever, get yeast infections. Eating coconut oil on a regular basis, as the Filipinos do, helps to keep yeast overgrowth at bay.

Assist digestive secretions. A major step in treating candidiasis is improving digestive secretions. Gastric hydrochloric acid, pancreatic enzymes, and bile all inhibit the overgrowth of yeasts and prevent its penetration into the surfaces of the small intestine. Decreased secretion of any of these components can lead to a proliferation of *C. albicans.*

Other conditions associated with low stomach acid include malabsorption, pernicious anemia, rosacea, eczema, iron deficiency anemia, food allergies, thyroid dysfunction, vitiligo, atrophic gastritis, helicobacter pylori infection of the stomach, and gastric cancer. Most holistic doctors have the materials to perform the Gastric Challenge Test to measure the amount of stomach acid you have.

Supplementation with hydrochloric acid (HCL betaine), pancreatic enzymes, and nutrients that improve bile flow are all crucial in treating chronic candidiasis. The *proteases* (pancreatic enzymes) are enzymes that break down proteins and are mostly responsible for keeping the small intestines free of parasites (yeasts, bacteria, protozoa, and worms). (A deficiency in proteases is also one of the reasons some people experience excessive hair breakage or loss of hair.) Supplementation should include HCL betaine, pancreatic enzymes, and a lipotropic formula to promote bile flow (the formula should include choline, methionine, and/or cysteine).

Support the immune system. A compromised immune system leads to yeast overgrowth and *C. albicans* infection promotes damage to the immune system. It's a vicious cycle. Tests can document immune dysfunction, but they are expensive. A practical (and free) evaluation is to look at your health history. A history of viral infections including colds and flu, outbreaks of cold sores or genital herpes, and prostatitis in men and vaginal infections in women are indicative of

In my practice, I have had a few clients that have had detox symptoms after the very first time they used the coconut oil. Although most [people] are able to use it by the tablespoon from the start, I have learned to start very ill and sensitive people on one teaspoon or less and work up from there. I have not had anyone so far that wasn't able to tolerate the four tablespoons [of coconut oil] per day if they work up to it. Even my people that have known histories of gallbladder and liver problems tolerate it very well. Also, digestive enzymes benefit everyone, and especially people with pancreas problems. [Coconut oil is] an effective therapy for yeasts, viruses, and bacteria, and die-off symptoms are a very real phenomenon.

—*Marie DeArmon*
Health Options Wellness Center,
Rogersville, MO

My scale tells me I lost five pounds in two weeks! I do have a little more energy, but because of die-off [symptoms] I also feel more tired [at times]. I am able to use my treadmill for 20 minutes a day and I do believe that virgin coconut oil has made that possible.

—*Lori*

immune dysfunction. This may be due to poor thyroid function. See chapter 4 for more information.

Supplementation with antioxidants, which include vitamins C and E, beta-carotene, selenium, and glutathione (found in abundance in vegetables), along with virgin coconut oil, can be very helpful in improving immune function.

Detoxify the liver. Drs. Michael Murray and Joseph Pizzorno say that improving liver health and promoting detoxification may be one of the most critical factors in the successful treatment of candidiasis. They note that damage to the liver is often an underlying factor in chronic candidiasis as well as chronic fatigue. Studies with mice have shown that even slight liver damage causes *C. albicans* to run rampant.[6] They recommend a three-day fast at the change of each season as part of the detoxification plan; you may want to choose a vegetable juice cleanse for your three-day fast. Phase II of The Coconut Diet outlines the liver cleanse program. Begin with the colon cleanse and then go to the liver cleanse, because if you cleanse your colon first, then you have a better chance of getting rid of toxins more quickly and efficiently when your liver starts releasing them.

Take probiotics. Probiotics, which are strains of beneficial intestinal flora such as *Lactobacillus acidophilus* and *Bactobacillus bifidum*, promote a healthy intestinal environment. Some of the very best probiotics are homeostatic soil organisms. (See Resources.) It is very important as you kill off the yeast to replace the good bacteria. Choose a good probiotic supplement as part of a wellness plan.

Take an antifungal compound. In addition to coconut oil (which has antifungal properties), you may benefit from taking a yeast-killing agent such as an herbal supplement that contains oregano and olive leaf.

Drink plenty of water. It is very important to drink plenty of water to flush your system as you kill off yeasts—aim for one quart of water for every 50 pounds of your weight. It will help to reduce die-off symptoms (discomfort as the yeast in your system dies) and promote weight loss and good hydration.

If you suspect you might suffer from candidiasis, W. G. Crook, M.D. has developed a questionnaire that you can fill out to determine the likelihood. (See page 101.)

THE HERXHEIMER REACTION

Be aware that as yeasts die, your symptoms may worsen for a short time or you may experience some adverse reactions such as headaches or diarrhea. Such reactions are known as the Herxheimer

I have only recently discovered coconut oil and want to relate how it caused a severe Herxheimer reaction. I've been battling a systemic candida yeast infection for more than 10 years. I [am in] the mutated (fungal) stage and it's the toughest thing I've ever had to deal with. I recently read research reports from Harvard and the University of Tennessee that this can be deadly and there are no pharmaceuticals for it that are effective. Candida yeast can overgrow in the gut under the right conditions until it mutates and becomes an invading pathogen, moves out of the gut and grows in mass in any part of the body. When it affects a vital organ, it can be deadly.

I've tried everything from conventional drugs to all the natural remedies including caprylic acid but have never experienced a die-off reaction as I did when I took the coconut oil and aerobic oxygen for about one week. I have subcutaneous masses on the scalp, face, buttocks, arms, and probably internally that I can't see. I applied the coconut [oil] heavily and would melt a large hunk in my mouth all during the day. My skin is starting to look better and I know from the reaction that it killed off a lot of candida.

The Herxheimer reaction is a welcome sign that you are doing something right. In cases where people are suffering with a chronic problem there may be a quick and somewhat adverse reaction. The "die-off effect," or Herxheimer reaction, refers to symptoms generated by a detoxification process. As the body begins to deal with dead microbes, one may experience a variety of detox symptoms. I am now recovering from the reaction and will start another round of coconut oil. [This oil] is something I will not be without for the rest of my life.

—*Tom*

reaction (die-off effect), which is the result of the rapid killing of microorganisms and absorption of large quantities of yeast toxins, cell particles, and antigens. Hang in there. Your health and weight loss will improve if you stick with the program.

I am a walking testimonial for the benefits of a low-carbohydrate, high-fat diet with regard to candida and cystitis. I used to purchase Monistat, two or three packages at a time. Now I use lots of coconut oil for cooking and eat plenty of coconut products such as fresh coconut, coconut flakes, and coconut milk. Coconut contains capric, caprylic, and lauric acid—all proven to kill candida, while leaving healthy intestinal flora intact. I was taking a long-term, broad-spectrum antibiotic for chronic cystitis for over two years and now it's been two years since I stopped refilling the prescription with no recurrence! By far the most remarkable transformation occurred when I started using coconut oil and simultaneously eliminated skim milk and all soy products from my diet. And I lost weight!

—*Laura*

DIGESTIVE DISORDERS

It is reported that about 95 million Americans suffer from some kind of digestive disorder. Americans spend more than $100 billion annually on digestive health care. This is over three times as much as is spent annually on weight loss, which is about $33 billion.

The major function of the gastrointestinal system is to break down and absorb nutrients. Without a well-functioning digestive system, essential nutrients that are necessary for maintaining proper weight and good health may not be absorbed adequately from the foods we eat, even if we are eating a healthy diet. This can lead to nutrient deficiencies, cravings, overeating, weight gain, and poor health.

When you are eating nutritious whole foods and avoiding refined carbohydrates, you should not gain weight. However, many people have switched to a healthy diet, and have even limited their carbohydrate intake, and still have problems losing weight. You may be one who suffers from poor digestion or a digestive disorder that prevents you from properly breaking down and utilizing your food. Even the best nutrition will go to waste if you are not able to process it.

When the body suffers from digestive disorders, it becomes difficult to digest fats. Thus, although it is important to eliminate unhealthy fats from our diet and switch to healthy fats like coconut oil and olive oil, we also need to make sure our digestive system can properly digest the fats we eat. Those with a poorly functioning pancreas have great difficulties in digesting fats. The pancreas produces enzymes (lipases, proteases, and amylases) that are required for breakdown and absorption of food. Lipases, along with bile, function in the breakdown of fats. Malabsorption (poor absorption) of fat and fat-soluble vitamins occurs when there is a deficiency of lipases.[7]

The digestive system is interrelated and one poorly functioning aspect of the system usually affects all the others. For example, the liver manufactures bile, which is important in the absorption of fats, oils, and fat-soluble vitamins. When the liver is impaired, and not able to produce enough bile, stools can become quite hard and difficult to pass. This affects the health of the colon and increases the reabsorption of toxins. Also, bile serves to keep the small intestine free from microorganisms such as *C. albicans* (yeasts), as previously noted in the candidiasis section.

Other digestive disorders include indigestion, irritable bowel syndrome (IBS), gastritis, diverticular disease, dysbiosis (altered bacterial flora), and constipation. More severe digestive disorders are known as inflammatory bowel disease (IBD) and include Crohn's disease and ulcerative colitis, which are characterized by an inflammatory reaction throughout the bowel. IBD sufferers usually experience bouts of diarrhea, cramping, and weight loss.

Whether or not you have been diagnosed with a digestive disorder, if you have trouble with digestion in any form—gas, bloating, flatulence or constipation to more severe problems such as those mentioned above—chances are that your organs of elimination need detoxifying and your digestive system needs some help. This is especially true as one ages.

The colon cleanse, liver cleanse, and other cleanses of The Coconut Diet were developed to help overcome these problems that affect digestive health and the ability to lose weight. They are a unique

I began taking virgin coconut oil after I read about it in *Woman's World* magazine. At the time I had a lot of problems with hypothyroid, fibromyalgia, IBS, candida, super dry skin, and skin rashes. I have stopped taking all meds for my gastrointestinal symptoms and my skin is now silky soft and smooth. I continue buying the virgin coconut oil (VCO) in larger and larger quantities. I recently finished the regimen of Fungal Defense [*Candida albicans* and yeast cleanse]. I am now taking the Primal Defense [homeostatic soil organisms]. I feel free of the *Candida albicans* (and constant yeast infections) for the first time in ages.

—*Michai*

part of The Coconut Diet and make it more effective than many other low-carb diets, along with the addition of coconut oil.

Coconut oil is one of the best fats to consume while trying to rebuild digestive health. For many years researchers have recognized that the medium-chain fatty acids (MCFAs) in coconut oil are digested differently than the longer-chain fatty acids found in today's refined vegetable oils. MCFAs are broken down first by enzymes in the saliva and gastric juices; therefore, enzymes from the pancreas are not needed as much.[8] Thus, people with digestive disorders have a greater ability to digest these smaller MCFAs in coconut oil. The body is able to convert MCFAs into energy instead of storing them in fat cells. Numerous studies have shown the weight loss effects of MCFAs (see chapter 3). The longer-chain fatty acids have a much greater tendency to be deposited in fat cells throughout the body.

As your body adjusts to coconut oil and good fats again, many digestive problems should improve. Those with more challenging digestive disorders, such as chronic constipation, should begin with a colon cleanse and follow the diet in Phase I. Follow the meal plan of Phase I or III for the additional weeks of Phase I, which are the Liver Cleanse, Gallbladder Cleanse, and Kidney Cleanse. (See chapter 7, "Phase II: Cleansing.")

FIBROMYALGIA AND CHRONIC FATIGUE SYNDROME

Fibromyalgia (FM) and chronic fatigue syndrome (CFS) have similar symptoms, with FM being characterized by musculoskeletal pain and CFS by fatigue. The exact cause of these illnesses is unknown and diagnosis is sometimes difficult. Many health professionals believe that a depressed immune system is the underlying cause of CFS with a virus such as Epstein-Barr or herpes or hypothyroid as a contributing factor. Sufferers describe feeling like a truck just ran over them. They experience constant muscle soreness and have very little energy to do anything. Even the thought of exercising seems overwhelming. This alone makes it difficult to lose weight. To screen yourself for this condition, see the Fibromyalgia Syndrome Questionnaire on page 107. To begin improving FM or CFS conditions, include the following:

- *Support your adrenal and thyroid glands.* Most fibromyalgia and chronic fatigue syndrome patterns involve exhausted adrenal glands and underactive thyroid. Studies show it is important to normalize blood sugar by eating foods low on the glycemic index, to avoid substances that tax the adrenals and thyroid such as caffeine (coffee, black tea, green tea, chocolate, and soda pop), alcohol, and sugar and include supplements that support the adrenal glands such as vitamin C, B_5, enzymes, and pantothenic acid. See chapter 4 for more information on thyroid support.
- *Eat a low-carb diet.* The Coconut Diet is ideal for FM and CFS sufferers since it is low in carbohydrates. High-carbohydrate foods should be completely avoided and replaced with lean proteins, vegetables, seeds, nuts, legumes, and healthy fats.
- *Include foods that are rich in magnesium.* Focus especially on foods rich in magnesium, since low magnesium levels are quite common in FM and CFS sufferers. Magnesium participates in more than 300 enzymatic reactions in the body, especially those that produce energy. Low magnesium levels mean low en-

ergy. Foods rich in magnesium include legumes, seeds, nuts, and green leafy vegetables. You may also need magnesium supplementation.[9]

- *Cleanse your body of toxins.* Cleansing is a very important part of correcting these conditions. I know firsthand. In my early 30s, I suffered from a devastating case of chronic fatigue syndrome that included chronic pain. I completely turned my health around through vegetable juicing, cleansing, and totally changing my diet. You can read my story of recovery at www.gococonuts.com. I recommend that if you suffer from either CFS or FM, that you start with Phase II (the cleansing programs) and follow the diet outlined in Phase I.
- *Take two to three tablespoons of virgin coconut oil each day.* If you read chapter 1, you know that the MCTs in coconut oil provide a

I have been on guaifenesin for fibromyalgia for over 3½ years. I've been using coconut oil for 1½ years. The coconut oil has been an important adjunct to my treatment. The protocol does work. I went from being severely disabled, walking with a cane (and shopping for an electric scooter) to working full time for my seasonal business.

—*Anne*

I had read about virgin coconut oil in *Woman's World* magazine. I ordered it for a sluggish thyroid and to see if it would help my fibromyalgia symptoms. I was disappointed after trying it the first day when I did not get any of the flushed feeling that I read about [on the coconut discussion group website]. I thought, "Maybe this will not help me either." This morning, however, after just three days of taking the virgin coconut oil, I got out of bed for the first time in years with no muscle aches or stiffness. It [the stiffness] is gone after just three days!

—*Tammy*

quick source of energy and stimulate the metabolism. Plus, the fatty acids in coconut oil can kill viruses such as Epstein-Barr, herpes, and giardia. With fewer viral organisms taxing the system, the immune system can function more efficiently. Thanks to coconut oil, I have received a number of reports from fibromyalgia sufferers who are living pain free and CFS sufferers who now have the energy to live a normal life.

UNDERACTIVE THYROID

Hypothyroidism is one of the reasons people on traditional low-carb diets cannot lose weight. The Coconut Diet is especially suited for people who have a hard time losing weight due to thyroid problems. See chapter 4 for more information.

EMOTIONAL EATING

Many times we eat food, not because we're hungry but because we are feeling emotional—sad, depressed, discouraged, bored, or anxious. At such times, that "little devil" on our shoulder says, "Yep, you're right! It's been a crummy day and you need some cheering up. You may as well eat the rest of that carton of ice cream or the double-chocolate cheesecake: You'll feel a lot better!"

Stress triggers a drop in serotonin levels, which can cause cravings for sweets and starches such as cookies, pasta, or breads. Women may be more susceptible to stress eating because of fluctuating hormones, and PMS can cause women to eat more junk food and sweets. These foods can help improve moods and induce happy memories or feelings, momentarily at least. Their lure has both chemical and emotional triggers. Some foods work on serotonin levels in the brain, producing a calming effect; they produce higher levels of serotonin, which is a little like "instant Prozac." Others work on an emotional level, reminding us of comfort and warmth from days of yore. But these "temporary fixes" have a price.

Ask yourself the following:

- Do I eat fattening foods when I'm bored or depressed to divert myself from bad moods?
- Which foods are most comforting for me?
- Which ones are calming?
- Which foods do I choose to eat when I'm stressed out or anxious?

Food is so powerfully connected to feelings that it sometimes seems impossible to consider various foods apart from their connection to emotions. There are many emotions attached to our favorite foods—the joy of celebrations, the pain of tragedies, happy moments, sad days, boredom, anxiety, and pleasure. Our favorite foods can evoke powerful emotions. They connect together a variety of associations that are difficult to separate—memories, emotions, and feelings. From infancy we have developed deep feelings about food, often buried in the subconscious. When we cried as babies, we were fed and the pain of hunger was replaced by a warm, full tummy. As children, food soothed emotional distress. As adults, we self-medicate our anxieties, hurts, fears, loneliness, and disappointments. Food is a reliable friend, consistent and dependable. It can be a surrogate for human contact and the bridge by which we form connections.

How many parties or social gatherings have you been to that didn't serve food? Food is the center of celebrations. Think about Thanksgiving, Christmas, Hanukkah, birthdays, the Fourth of July, weddings, dating, and social gatherings. I'll bet you have a long list of "celebration foods" you enjoy at such times. We all have positive emotions regarding our favorite foods served on special occasions. Most of us also have a list of "comfort foods" and that we turn to when we're ill or emotionally distressed. When the going gets tough, we often gravitate to the feel-good foods we remember fondly from our youth—everything from macaroni and cheese to mashed potatoes and gravy, hot bread and butter, chocolate chip cookies and ice cream sundaes.

If your boyfriend dumps you, grilled fish and squash probably won't cut it. If you get fired from your job, split pea soup and salad probably won't be what you order for lunch. What do you eat when bad things happen? If you're like most of us, you're going to go for foods that are emotionally comforting. And those are usually the foods you grew up eating as a child.

Many have grown up on brand-name products that have little in common with the whole, natural foods they were processed from. And most of us prefer these foods. Even for those who have eaten a whole-foods diet for years, there is still, somewhere back in the sub-liminal recesses of our emotions, fond memories of such things as steaming bowls of canned noodle soup served with a sandwich made of soft, snowy white bread grilled in margarine and stuffed with melted, orange-colored cheese. Mothers, who were either frazzled by overwork, or seduced by the concept of convenience, served high-carb processed foods with love, and although they may have been anything but wholesome, in the subconscious they are still desirable.

But what is the price of unhealthy comfort foods or simple-pleasure indulgences? Many of us could say weight gain for one; poor health for another. Unfortunately, all who grew up on a diet of brand-name foods that are high in refined carbs and sugars have some major rethinking and attitude adjustment in store if we wish to successfully adopt a healthy diet that will promote weight management.

We've also grown up with the "bigger is better" mentality in this country. It's the "super-size me" slogan that's become so popular today in everything from all-you-can-eat buffets to Big Macs and colossal shakes. We've come to believe we didn't get our money's worth unless it's a large portion. So when we're dealing with emotions, we not only want that favorite indulgence, we want it in a large size.

It is never easy to make a major change, even when our better sense says this is the best program for weight loss and good health. No mat-ter how convinced or motivated we are there is still a little voice, some-where in our inner depths, screaming, "I want sugar-frosted breakfast flakes!" and no matter what foods we choose as a temporary "fix" for our screaming emotions, the positive effects are only momentary. In the end, they set us up for real depression about our weight, low en-ergy, and ill health. It's not always easy to make changes, but if we con-sider that making no change can mean a lifetime of being overweight, unhealthy, and tired, the decision to change becomes easier.

THE RIGHT RESPONSE: JOHN'S STORY

I'd like to ask you a question: Are you discouraged, angry, or depressed about all the things you can't eat on a low-carb diet? If you aren't now, you may be by the time you have finished Cherie's lists of "foods to avoid" in part II. If you can no longer eat everything you want, be aware that frustration is normal. In the midst of negative emotions, change can happen; it's a matter of choosing the right responses.

When I, John, was diagnosed with hypoglycemia, I was initially relieved and excited to finally find out about the cause of my fatigue, irritability, and headaches. Then, as I learned about what I would have to give up eating and drinking to feel better, my enthusiasm and excitement quickly gave in to downright panic. I had a genuine concern that I'd never be able to let go of the foods and beverages that had become so much a part of my life. It's now funny to think about how matter-of-fact the doctor was as he read off the list of what I could and couldn't eat—never, ever again! My first thought was to chain myself up, but in actuality, I realized I had to figure out a way I could make the new diet work.

You may be dealing with frustration about the foods you need to give up to lose weight. Actually emotional attachments to certain foods and eating to deal with various emotions are key reasons people don't succeed on weight loss programs. Be aware that you can choose to make wise choices and overcome emotional eating. I did, and it paid off. The following guidelines can help you make the right responses to food.

Choice Responses

One of the easiest ways to be effective when it comes to changing our eating habits is to associate the results of our actions with the outcome. In questioning individuals who have been successful in losing weight, one characteristic stands out. These individuals were able to imagine the relationship between their present choices and the effect those choices would have on their diet program. A default response, as opposed to a choice response, is when an individual has only one automatic response in a situation and can't seem to get beyond that, even when the outcome is adverse. From time to time, many of us respond in this manner. But if we are rarely able to get beyond the default response, regardless of the outcome, it is time to assess our behavior and set new goals for change.

FINDING A SOLUTION

Ask yourself the following questions when you're tempted to emotionally eat or go on food binges:

- What am I really feeling?
- Can I just be with this feeling?
- If I eat this fattening food, or go on a sugar binge, what will it cost me in the long run?
- What's really important to me now?
- Is there a better way to take care of myself both emotionally and physically?
- What can I give myself right now that won't cost me my power?
- How can I nurture myself right now without hurting myself?
- If I were a child right now, how would I really like to be comforted?
- What can I do today that will make me feel good tomorrow?
- How can I reward myself with things that are good for me?

DEVELOP A LIST OF HEALTHY REWARDS

What rewards can you think of that won't hurt your body? Following are a few suggestions:

- Call a friend.
- Take a walk.
- Watch a favorite movie.
- Take a hot bath by candlelight with your favorite music and a cup of tea.

- Work out and work away your worries; exercise can help—it raises endorphins and other "feel good" hormones.
- Form a list of healthy foods for rewards.

A PLAN OF ACTION

- Get a journal and write about your food cravings; writing about the cravings can be helpful.
- Let your emotions speak, rather than suppressing them; write about them.
- Ask your cravings questions. You may be surprised at what you hear. The point is to hear them out and find out what your real need is.
- Food suppresses emotions; allow your urges to be heard and understood.
- Think about a trim, healthy person you admire. How do you think that person would handle a food-binge urge?
- Learn to have fun without food.
- Cultivate personal power.
- Increase nurturing life experiences that can help you get beyond junk food and comfort-food eating.
- Accept your emotions, rather than stuffing them or shutting them down.
- Allow your emotions to come up and let them go.
- Courageously face painful emotions without stuffing them or covering them up.
- Invite nurturing people into your life.
- Cultivate self-loving experiences.
- Practice stress reduction.

SETTING GOALS FOR DIETARY CHANGE

If you find yourself motivated to eat the wrong foods because of an emotional response, I suggest you go through the following process to keep yourself from sabotaging your weight loss efforts.

1. Get a plan clearly in mind about what you are going to do the next time you are tempted to eat the foods you know aren't on The Coconut Diet's list of foods you can enjoy—foods that will sabotage your weight loss plans.

2. Associate your actions with the outcome of your choices. Be as graphic as you can and try to actually feel what you would experience physically if you ate the things that you shouldn't eat. Or, if you experience no adverse physical sensations, think about how this food might impact your weight loss. How will you feel when you step on the scale and see you've gained a pound or two?

3. Picture the foods that are detrimental to your weight loss program with a very negative symbol such as the words "rat poison" written above them or any other negative association that will really turn you off.

4. Associate the foods that are part of your weight loss program with positive thoughts such as "Mineral water with a slice of lemon is a great party drink! It's better for me than alcohol and tastes just as good."

5. Develop a list of "right choice" comfort foods that you can turn to when you're emotionally down and make these the accepted foods for celebrations. Make sure you have some of these foods on hand at all times so you aren't tempted to go out for ice cream or nachos when your emotions are screaming for comforting food or you feel like celebrating.

6. The next time you go out to dinner or prepare a special meal at home, and you're tempted to throw caution to the wind and splurge, remember that what you eat will impact your weight loss. Think about how you'll feel the next morning when you step on the scale or when you reflect on what you did. You've embarked on a special mission to lose weight.

7. If you splurge, don't punish yourself. Start over the very next meal with a positive plan to make wise choices in the future. And no matter what, never succumb to the temptation of throwing the whole plan out because you've "blown it" a time or two. Just pick yourself up "and get back in the race."[10]

CANDIDA QUESTIONNAIRE

There are different point scores for each question below. Note the points and add them up. The score evaluation is at the end of the quiz.

Section 1: History	Point Score
1. Have you taken tetracycline or other antibiotics for acne for one month or longer?	25
2. Have you at any time in your life taken other "broad-spectrum" antibiotics for respiratory, urinary, or other infections for two months or longer, or in short courses four or more times in a one-year period?	20
3. Have you ever taken a broad-spectrum antibiotic (even a single course)?	6
4. Have you at any time in your life been bothered by persistent prostatitis, vaginitis, or other problems affecting your reproductive organs?	25
5. Have you been pregnant one time?	3
Two or more times?	5
6. Have you taken birth control pills for six months to two years?	8
For more than two years?	15
7. Have you taken prednisone or other cortisone-type drugs for two weeks or less?	6
For more than two weeks?	15
8. Does exposure to perfumes, insecticides, fabric shop odors, and other chemicals provoke mild symptoms?	5
Moderate to severe symptoms?	20

Continued

9. Are your symptoms worse on damp, muggy days or
   in moldy places?   20

10. Have you had athlete's foot, ringworm, "jock itch,"
    or other chronic infections of the skin or nails?
    Mild to moderate?   10
    Severe or persistent?   20

11. Do you crave sugar?   10

12. Do you crave breads?   10

13. Do you crave alcoholic beverages?   10

14. Does tobacco smoke really bother you?   10

Total Score for section 1 _____

Section 2: Major Symptoms

For each of your symptoms below, enter the appropriate figure in the point score column.

If symptom is occasional or mild   score 3 points
If symptom is frequent and/or moderately severe   score 6 points
If a symptom is severe and/or disabling   score 9 points

                                                          Score

1. Fatigue or lethargy   _____

2. Feeling of being drained   _____

3. Poor memory   _____

4. Feeling "spacey" or "unreal"   _____

5. Depression _____

6. Numbness, burning, or tingling _____

7. Muscle aches _____

8. Muscle weakness or paralysis _____

9. Pain and/or swelling in joints _____

10. Abdominal pain _____

11. Constipation _____

12. Diarrhea _____

13. Bloating _____

14. Persistent vaginal itch _____

15. Persistent vaginal burning _____

16. Prostatitis _____

17. Impotence _____

18. Loss of sexual desire _____

19. Endometriosis _____

20. Cramping and other menstrual irregularities _____

21. Premenstrual tension _____

22. Spots in front of eyes _____

23. Erratic vision _____

Total score for section 2 _____

Section 3: Other Symptoms

For each of the symptoms below, enter the appropriate figure in the point score column.

If symptom is occasional or mild	score 1 point
If symptom is frequent and/or moderately severe	score 2 points
If a symptom is severe and/or disabling	score 3 points

Score

1. Drowsiness   _____

2. Irritability   _____

3. Lack of coordination   _____

4. Inability to concentrate   _____

5. Frequent mood swings   _____

6. Headache   _____

7. Dizziness/loss of balance   _____

8. Pressure above ears, feeling of head swelling and tingling   _____

9. Itching   _____

10. Rashes   _____

11. Heartburn   _____

12. Indigestion   _____

13. Belching and intestinal gas   _____

14. Mucus in stools   _____

15. Hemorrhoids   _____

16. Dry mouth   _____

17. Rash or blisters in mouth   _____

18. Bad breath   _____

19. Joint swelling or arthritis   _____

20. Nasal congestion or discharge   _____

21. Postnasal drip   _____

22. Nasal itching   _____

23. Sore or dry throat   _____

24. Cough   _____

25. Pain or tightness in chest   _____

26. Wheezing or shortness of breath   _____

27. Urinary urgency or frequency   _____

28. Burning on urination   _____

29. Failing vision   _____

30. Burning or tearing of eyes   _____

31. Recurrent infections or fluid in ears   _____

32. Ear pain or deafness   _____

Total score for section 3   _____

Total score for section 1 _____

Total score for section 2 _____

Total score for section 3 _____

Total score for all sections _____

	Women	**Men**
Yeast-connected health problems are almost certainly present	>180	>140
Yeast-connected health problems are probably present	120–180	90–140
Yeast-connected health problems are possibly present	60–119	40–89
Yeast-connected health problems are less likely to be present	<60	<40

This questionnaire is adapted from W. G. Crook, M.D., *The Yeast Connection*. Although the Candida Questionnaire can help determine your condition, ultimately the best method for diagnosing candidiasis is a clinical evaluation by a physician knowledgeable about yeast-related illness.

FIBROMYALGIA SYNDROME QUESTIONNAIRE

Please score each symptom as follows:

          3 points = always
          2 points = often
          1 point = sometimes
          0 points = never

Symptoms   **Score**

Major criteria

1. Widespread pain   _____

2. Sleep disturbance   _____

3. Fatigue   _____

4. Morning stiffness   _____

Minor criteria

5. Weight gain   _____

6. Anxiety   _____

7. Irritable bowel syndrome   _____

8. Headaches   _____

9. Cold hands and/or feet (Raynaud's disease)   _____

10. Dry mouth or eyes   _____

11. Depression   _____

Continued

12. Numbness or tingling _____

13. Allergies _____

14. Hypoglycemia _____

15. Excessive mucus _____

16. Fluid retention _____

17. PMS _____

18. Painful menstruation _____

19. Adversely affected by heat or cold _____

20. Adversely affected by weather changes _____

21. Family history of similar symptoms _____

22. Tinnitus (ringing in the ears) _____

23. Dizziness/vertigo _____

24. Tachycardia _____

25. Short-term memory problems _____

26. Brain fog _____

27. Flu-like symptoms _____

28. Sensitivity to smells, light, sound, and vibrations _____

29. Muscle twitches _____

30. Ringing in ears _____

Total score _____

Contributing Factors

1. Sexual or physical abuse in childhood   _____

2. Recurring family stress regarding symptoms   _____

The first four points are fairly indicative of fibromyalgia (FM). If you scored 2 or 3 on at least three of the four major criteria, and 2 or 3 on five or more minor criteria, you could have FM. To determine whether or not you have FM, see a physician who specializes in the treatment of this condition.

PART II

The Coconut Diet

Chapter 6/Phase I

The 21-Day Weight Loss Kickoff

Welcome to *the most* exciting low-carb weight loss program available. You're about to experience weight loss with ease, taste satisfaction, and plenty of fabulous food choices. You're off to a great start with the 21-Day Weight Loss Kickoff! And, like so many dieters, you, too, will be amazed at how you feel—with improved energy, loss of sugar cravings, and better sleep.

Phase I is the strictest phase of The Coconut Diet, and it offers the greatest results. For the first 21 days you will eat healthy lean protein such as chicken, turkey, fish, beef, eggs, cheese, and nuts with lots of nonstarchy vegetables, leafy greens, and good fats. Grain products such as bread, bagels, muffins, rolls, buns, crackers, rice cakes, cereals, rice, pasta, and pizza and even whole grains such as oatmeal, quinoa, and barley will be avoided. Sweets are off the list too—no cakes, cookies, pies, ice cream, doughnuts, or candy along with most fruit and starchy vegetables such as potatoes, corn, and acorn squash.

If you think you will have nothing exciting left to eat, you'll be happily surprised. The Coconut Diet offers delicious foods and recipes that are part of the 21-day meal plan, which includes Vegetable Quiche On-the-Go, Crispy Coconut Chicken Salad, Thai Coconut Salmon, and the Low-Carb Coconut Smoothie along with dozens of other mouth-watering recipes for you to choose from that will keep your taste buds satisfied. And coconut oil will help curb your cravings for sweets, bread, and starches, too.

You can choose good carbohydrates from a wide variety of brightly colored vegetables rich in antioxidants and other important vitamins and minerals that will support your immune system. Most of these foods you can eat as often as you like and as much as you want. Lean meats, poultry, fish, eggs, cheese, and nuts will give your body the protein it needs. You can eat these foods in moderate portions.

Healthy fats, especially coconut oil, will help to satisfy your hunger faster and more completely. Coconut oil makes this program uniquely successful in that it helps boost the body's metabolism. This oil burns quickly, much like kindling in a fireplace. It helps curb cravings, especially for sweets, and keeps hunger at bay. You will consume two to three tablespoons of coconut oil per day. You may also include olive oil and small amounts of butter.

This is not a diet of deprivation, but one of enjoyment. With three meals per day and two snacks, you should not feel hungry or deprived. Best of all, you will learn a new style of eating that you can follow for the rest of your life. To keep track of your foods and supplements use the Daily Food Log (page 152).

Within days of starting this program, you should enjoy more energy and feel healthier. Some physical ailments may simply disappear. One improvement that is typically mentioned is a lessening of fatigue. In fact, people often report great energy surges. Many women note a significant reduction in PMS symptoms. Joint problems improve for many. And scores of people who have suffered from low thyroid function experienced exciting improvements.

The Coconut Diet is not only enjoyable—it's easy. You're not being asked to measure food or count carbs—just choose from the lists of low-carbohydrate foods you can eat, and don't eat the foods on the "avoid" lists.

Low-carb eating will give your body a chance to deal with issues of insulin resistance brought on by eating too many of the wrong carbs, which are primarily the refined and processed ones. When you no longer experience swings in blood sugar, it will be easier to control cravings for sweets and other high-carbohydrate foods. As a result, you will lose weight faster.

At the end of Phase I, you should have lost your cravings for sweets, bread, and starches. As a result, your body should be far less

I started taking virgin coconut oil about four weeks ago and have gone from 248 pounds down to 222. I eat a high-protein, high-fat, low-carb diet and I walk six to nine miles a day. Before I started using three tablespoons of virgin coconut oil, I had reached a plateau for five and a half months, only losing six pounds. [Coconut oil] is the only thing I've changed [in my diet].

—*Leia*

When I started [taking coconut oil], I weighed 316 pounds and wore a size 52 pant. When I got on the scale this morning, I weighed 256 pounds for a total weight loss of 60 pounds. I'm now in a size 44 pant. The weight is virtually falling off with minimal exercise—maybe a couple of walks of 30 to 60 minutes a week. To me the secret of weight loss is no processed white stuff, lots of quality oils and fats, and an adequate intake of protein.

—*Chuck*

resistant to insulin and your blood sugar should be more stable. Best of all, you will be living a lifestyle that will help you prevent serious diseases such as heart disease, cancer, and diabetes.

EXERCISE AND WEIGHT LOSS

Although exercise is not a specific element of The Coconut Diet, it is a great way to boost metabolism, speed up weight loss, and improve overall health. Exercising will not only help you burn fat and tone and build muscle, it will help you increase your metabolism. Boosting your metabolism makes weight loss occur faster and more easily. You'll also enjoy a mental boost (it increases endorphins), it enhances relaxation, and helps you sleep better; it's similar to the effects of an antidepressant. Additionally, women who lose estrogen increasingly with the onset of menopause can combat bone loss, depression, and breast cancer by exercising regularly.

What kind of exercise helps? Experts say we should combine aerobic exercise and strength training (weights) if we want to burn fat and tone up. Everything from walking, swimming, biking, step aerobics to weight lifting is great. If you can't get outside or to the gym, consider trying a book and video series using hand weights called *Walk Away the Pounds* that you can use in your own home (see Resources). Pick the fitness routine that's right for you and stick with it no matter what. Aim for a minimum of three times per week.

The mini-trampoline (also known as a rebounder) is helpful for the lymphatic system and to help clear clogged lymph nodes; it's also very good for the internal organs. Jumping on the mini-trampoline is a great form of exercise that you can do at home any time. (See Resources.)

Another great machine is the lymphasizer (aerobic oxygenator or swing machine), which provides gentle massage as it oxygenates muscles, tissues, and organs. The movement is similar to a fish swimming. It also helps move the lymph along so it doesn't stagnate. And it promotes weight loss. If you are not able to do a lot of exercise right now, or you want to supplement your exercise program, this machine may be the ticket. You just lie on the floor with each ankle in a groove and turn the machine on. It does the rest for you. My husband and I use our lymphasizer frequently. (See Resources.)

SLEEP FOR WEIGHT LOSS

According to the National Sleep Foundation, 74 percent of Americans have trouble sleeping at least a few nights a week. This not only can make us tired, grumpy, and forgetful, new research suggests that chronic sleep loss can make us gain weight. A recent study of 8,274 Japanese children found that those who slept less than 8 hours a night were nearly three times as likely to be obese as those who slept 10 hours or more. Sleep deprivation can increase cortisol levels, re-

> I've been on virgin coconut oil less than a week and I'm already feeling better—sleeping better, less cravings, skin looks better, less breakouts. Can this be so? Seems too good to be true!
>
> —*Teresa*

duce glucose tolerance, and diminish thyroid hormones, which can contribute to insulin resistance and a sluggish metabolism. With less sleep we can become more of a fat storer and less of a calorie burner.[1]

Numerous dieters have reported that adding coconut oil to their diet has helped them get a good night's sleep. But be aware that consuming coconut oil less than four to five hours before bedtime may be too energizing and keep you awake. Other helpful hints for sleeping well include a few drops of lavender oil on your pillow and a cup of chamomile tea or other herbal nighttime tea before bed. Replenishing minerals such as calcium and magnesium along with vitamin C can be very helpful if you are deficient. There is an herbal supplement (Tranquilnite) that can help you sleep more soundly. A drop of Rescue Remedy rubbed on your wrist just before bed is especially helpful when traveling or under stress. Both can be found at health food stores. Also, correcting low thyroid function and balancing blood sugar can be helpful in correcting sleep disorders. Most important, try not to think of anything that will produce anxious thoughts as you near bedtime. Your mind could keep ruminating on the subject long after you wish to go to sleep. Stress reduction techniques such as prayer or meditation could be helpful.

FOODS YOU CAN EAT

Servings Per Day
- Animal protein: four to six ounces per meal
- Eggs: no more than two per day
- Fruit: One or two servings per day

- Legumes: One or two one-cup servings per week
- Nuts: seeds, nut butters: 24 small nuts such as almonds; six large nuts such as macadamia; one teaspoon nut or seed butter
- Sweetener: small amount of low-carb healthy sweetener
- Vegetables: Unlimited

Animal Proteins

Choose healthy, antibiotic-free (preferably organic) lean cuts of meat and poultry in moderate portions; choose wild-caught fish.

Beef
    Lean cuts of meat are best, such as: flank, lean beef bacon (limit 2 slices), New York sirloin, tenderloin, top round
Bison (buffalo)
Eggs
Elk
Fish of all types
Lamb
Poultry
    Chicken: skinless breast and thighs are best
    Cornish game hens
    Turkey: skinless is best
    Turkey bacon (limit 2 slices)
Venison

Dairy

Choose antibiotic-free (preferably organic) dairy products.

Cheese
    Best choices are: feta, goat cheese, Gruyère, mozzarella, ricotta, Swiss
Cream (in small amounts)

Beverages

Green tea (omit if you have taxed thyroid or adrenal)
Herbal tea (hot and iced)

Mineral water with lemon or lime or unsweetened cranberry concentrate for flavor

Vegetable juices

Cereal Grass
Wild rice (often thought of as a grain)

Eggs
Choose cage free, preferably organic.

Fats and Oils
Butter

Coconut oil (virgin is best)

Olive oil (extra virgin is best)

Fruit
Avocado (1 small to medium California)

Cranberry

Lemon

Lime

Tomatoes

Milk
Almond milk

Coconut milk

Rice milk

Nuts and Nut Butters; Seeds and Seed Butters
(Try not to eat more than the suggested serving per day. If you combine nuts and seeds, keep the serving size in mind because nuts and seeds have carbohydrates as well as protein and fat.)

Almond (no more than 2 dozen)

Almond butter (1 teaspoon)

Brazil nut (no more than 6)

Cashew (no more than 6)

Cashew butter (1 teaspoon)

Hazelnut (no more than 24)
Hazelnut butter (1 teaspoon)
Macadamia (no more than 12)
Macadamia nut butter (1 teaspoon)
Peanut (actually not a nut—a legume) (no more than 24 small)
Peanut butter (1 teaspoon)
Pecan halves (no more than 12)
Pine nut (no more than 24)
Pistachio (no more than 24)
Pumpkin seed (no more than 2 tablespoons)
Sesame seed (no more than 2 tablespoons)
Sunflower seed (no more than 2 tablespoons)
Tahini (sesame seed butter) (1 teaspoon)
Walnut halves (no more than 12)

Note: You may have two dehydrated seed crackers per day in place of nuts or seeds; most of them also have vegetable fiber added. Seed crackers are dehydrated and considered a raw food; they are made without grains. Some health food stores carry them, or you can make them in a dehydrator. Almost all raw food recipe books have recipes for dehydrated crackers.

Sweeteners
Birch sugar (xylitol)
Lo Han
Stevia

Vegetables and Legumes

Artichoke
Asparagus
Bamboo shoot
Beans
Beet and beet greens
Bok choi
Broccoflower
Broccoli
Broccoli rabe
Broccolini
Brussels sprouts
Cabbage: Chinese, green, red, Savoy
Carrot
Cassava
Cauliflower
Celeriac
Celery

Chard
Chayote
Collard
Cucumber
Dandelion greens
Eggplant
Endive
Fennel
Jicama
Kale
Kohlrabi
Legumes (dried beans, lentils, split peas)
Lettuce
All varieties, which include: bibb/Boston, greenleaf, iceberg, redleaf, romaine, spring greens/mesclun
Mushrooms
All varieties, which include: oyster, portobello, shiitake, straw, whole button
Mustard greens
Okra
Onion
Parsley

Pea pods
Peas
Peppers: green, purple, red, yellow
Radicchio
Radish
Rutabaga
Sauerkraut
Scallion
Sorrel
Spinach
Sprouts
Squash: hubbard, spaghetti, summer/yellow, zucchini
Taro
Tomatillo
Tomato (considered a vegetable; actually a fruit, classified a berry)
All varieties, which include: cherry, plum, red (includes beefsteak), Roma, sun-dried, yellow pear
Turnip
Water chestnut
Watercress

Don't Forget Your Vitamins

When you're cutting back on food in general, and certain foods in particular, such as fruits and grains, it's important to fill in the gaps with a good multivitamin capsule. Be aware that not all supplements are high quality. You'll pay a little more for a natural high-quality supplement, and it's worth it.

CHOOSING THE BEST

When you choose animal protein, vegetables, legumes, fats, oils, and beverages, you want to choose the healthiest. If your body is well fed with a nutrient-rich diet, you will crave less and desire to eat less. In some cases, you may need to shop at a health food store. Shopping carefully is well worth the work because the goal of The Coconut Diet is not just weight loss; it's also improving your health.

Animal Protein

Choose free-range, grass-fed beef, whenever possible. CLA (conjugated linoleic acid) is mostly found in grass-fed dairy cow and beef products. The body cannot produce CLA; we must get it from our food. CLA has been shown to promote weight loss. See page 50 for more information.

Whenever possible, shop for antibiotic-free and preferably organically raised lamb and poultry. The growth hormones injected into factory-farm-raised animals cause them to gain weight. After all, fattening animals quickly to get them to market means more dollars for the vendors. But what does it mean for consumers? These hormones are not healthful and it is best to avoid them.

Eggs are an excellent protein source. They contain all eight essential amino acids and are a rich source of essential fatty acids. They also contain considerably more lecithin (a fat emulsifier) than cholesterol. They are also rich in sulfur and glutathione.

Natural foods markets such as Whole Foods and Wild Oats and many independent health food stores as well as local farmers markets have grass-fed or naturally raised beef, lamb, buffalo, and poultry. Also, look for eggs from chickens that are raised cage-free, without hormones, and fed an organic diet. And finally, buy organic dairy products such as cheese, milk, and cream whenever it is available.

When it comes to fish, buy wild-caught fish as much as possible. Farm-raised fish get by almost as poorly as factory farm animals.

They are often given antibiotics, raised penned in crowded pools, and not fed their customary marine diet. Hence, they do not have the essential fatty acids that wild-caught fish offer, which are so important for our health.

Quality lean protein is important for overall health and weight management. It stimulates the production of glucagon, a hormone that functions opposite insulin. Glucagon stabilizes blood sugar levels and provides brain fuel by signaling the body to release stored energy. When synchronized, insulin and glucagon create a stable hormonal system.

Keep in mind that you can get too much animal protein, however, which is taxing for the kidneys and can contribute to over-acidity in the system. That is why it is best to limit portion sizes between four and six ounces.

When it comes to animal fat, fish is a good source of omega-3 fatty acids, especially the fatty coldwater fish such as salmon, mackerel, and trout. Animal fat should be kept to a minimum. Animals are higher on the food chain and tend to store toxins more in the fat than the muscle. Though choosing organically raised animal products is far superior to factory-farm-raised animals that are grown in crowded, unhealthy conditions and given antibiotics and hormones, environmental toxins will be still stored in the animal's fat.

Beverages

Green tea is especially helpful for weight loss. Not only is it rich in antioxidants such as catechins and other polyphenols that protect us against inflammation, cancer, and other ailments, it is also a *thermogenic.* Thermogenesis means the production of heat, which revs up your metabolism. Most of the thermogenic action in green tea is due to epigallocatechin gallate (EGCG), a potent polyphenol. EGCG also appears to increase the effectiveness of weight loss supplements such as 5HTP and tyrosine.[2] For this reason, I recommend green tea as part of your daily meal plan. Strive for at least one cup of green tea per day. Avoid green tea, however, if you are caffeine sensitive, or have low adrenal or thyroid function or hypoglycemia; a cup of green tea has about one third of the caffeine found in a cup of coffee. When choosing green and herbal tea, look for the healthiest—organically grown teas. Unbleached tea bags are better choices over bleached.

Sparkling mineral water that is naturally carbonated, rather than commercially gassed, is the best choice, such as S. Pellegrino and Apollinaris.

Freshly made vegetable juices from organic produce is always the healthiest. When choosing canned or bottled juice such as V-8 juice, choose low sodium and organic, if available.

Drink at least eight to ten 8-ounce glasses of water per day. Purified water is best.

Fats and Oils

The best oils and fat for food preparation are virgin coconut oil, extra-virgin olive oil, and butter. It is best to choose organic when it comes to all three.

Consume two to three tablespoons of virgin coconut oil per day. Be choosy when it comes to coconut oil. Many commercial-grade coconut oils are made from *copra*, which means the dried kernel (meat) of the coconut. If standard copra is used as a starting material, the unrefined coconut oil extracted from copra is not suitable for human consumption and must be refined. This is because most copra is dried under the sun in the open air in very unsanitary conditions where it is exposed to insects and molds. Though producers may start with organic coconuts and even label their coconut oil organic, the end product of some brands is refined, bleached, and deodorized. High heat and chemical solvents are used in this process.

Virgin coconut oil made by hand produces a noticeable difference in taste, smell (more fragrant), color (whiter), and texture than oil made with standard copra. Traditionally made oil, which is known as virgin coconut oil, is far superior in every way. Although more costly, this oil is well worth it. (See Resources.)

I am one of those people who increased the dosage of virgin coconut oil to seven tablespoons per day and along with that had acupuncture once or twice a week for 10 sessions. I lost around 3 kilos [about 6½ pounds]. The incredible thing was that I never felt hungry, so losing weight was easy. I also noticed warmth in my feet and hands.

—*Michelle*

Olive oil is called *virgin* if it is extracted by means of pressure from millstones. Virgin olive oil is not treated with heat or chemicals. Batches of olives are pressed more than once to produce numerous batches of oil. The first pressing is the most flavorful and has the least acidity. The first cold pressing also has the highest amount of fatty acids and polyphenols (antioxidants). Olive oils from the Mediterranean, and particularly Spain, are the highest in antioxidants. The very best choice is extra-virgin, cold pressed olive oil that is organically grown in the Mediterranean.

Raw, cultured butter from dairy cows that have been raised naturally and grass-fed is the best choice. It's also rich in vitamin A and CLA, when it comes from grass-fed cows. Use butter more sparingly than the oils.

Fruit, Vegetables, and Legumes

Fruit. One of the best fruits is avocado. (Yes, avocado is a fruit.) It is an excellent source of essential fatty acids, glutathione (a powerful antioxidant), and a source of protein. It contains more potassium than bananas, which are off the list until you reach your weight loss goals, making them an excellent choice for heart disorders. Most fruit is off the list for the first three weeks, except for tomatoes and a little cranberry concentrate and lemon and lime juice to flavor beverages and salad dressings.

Vegetables. Most vegetables are on the list of allowed foods. You should eat lots of them, because they're packed with satisfying health-promoting nutrients. Eat lots of salads, sprouts, vegetable sticks, sea vegetables, and steamed vegetables. Avoid baked vegetables as much as possible, because the sugar content is highest in these. High-starch vegetables such as potatoes, yams, corn, and acorn squash are off the list. If you are dining out or it's a special occasion and you just can't resist a potato, the best choice is red potatoes (less carbs). If you do succumb to a baked potato, which is very high in carbs, eat it with fat like sour cream or butter. This will help to slow down the rate at which sugar enters your bloodstream.

Legumes (dried beans, lentils, and split peas) should be limited. The outer casing of legumes (fiber) does slow down the rate at which sugar enters your bloodstream. Limit beans, lentils, and split peas to no more than one or two 1-cup servings a week for the first three weeks.

Organic produce. Choose organic produce as often as possible to avoid toxic pesticides. In 1995 the USDA (United States Department of Agriculture) tested nearly 7,000 fruit and vegetable samples and detected residues of 65 different pesticides, with two out of three samples containing pesticide residue.

Plants absorb nutrients from the soil; they also take up pesticides. Healthy soil is rich in minerals and alive with microorganisms. Pesticides kill these much-needed microorganisms, and chemical fertilizers do not replenish the soil in any manner close to traditional composting and other natural practices that nourish soil.

The quality of protein in grains and vegetables is related to the amount of nitrogen in the soil. When there is a lot of nitrogen present, plants increase protein production and decrease carbohydrate synthesis. When the metabolic protein requirements are satisfied, the remaining protein produced is stored in the form of protein that contains fewer essential amino acids. The result of high levels of nitrogen, as found in conventional chemical fertilizers, is an increase in the amount of protein but a reduction in the quality of the protein. Organically managed soils release nitrogen in smaller amounts over a longer time period than conventional fertilizers. As a result, the quality of protein from organic crops is better in terms of human nutrition.[3]

While organic foods are always the best option in terms of avoiding pesticides, studies also show they are higher in nutrient content. In a 2001 study published in the *Journal of Alternative and Complementary Medicine,* on average, organic produce contained 27 percent more vitamin C, 21 percent more iron, and 29 percent more magnesium than conventional produce, and all 21 minerals compared in the study were higher in the organic produce.[4]

The more nutrient-rich foods you eat, the more your body will be satisfied and cravings will diminish. In this respect, organic produce is helpful for weight loss. But the most important reason to choose organically grown food is your health.

Salt

The best salt is sea salt or Celtic salt, also known as gray salt. Whole sea salt has a mineral profile that is similar to blood. Regular table salt is a highly refined product and therefore undesirable. When salt is processed, minerals are removed and what remains is primarily sodium chloride. Anticaking chemicals, potassium oxide, iodine, and dextrose (sugar) are added to make table salt. It is possible that some people tend to overeat salty foods because their bodies are craving the minerals that have been refined out of the salt. Too much salt can promote water retention and cause weight gain.

Spice Up Your Meals!

Black pepper, cayenne, ginger, and turmeric all have been shown to induce thermogenesis, which means they help the body metabolize fat. I've incorporated these spices often in the recipes, but you can add them as often as you like to any dish. Not only will you add great flavor and assist your body in burning fat, you'll help prevent some diseases such as cancer.

Sweeteners

The three low-carb healthy sweeteners that produce the best results are stevia, birch sugar (xylitol), and Lo Han Guo. (See page 23 for more information.)

FOODS TO AVOID

The foods in the "avoid" section should be completely omitted for three weeks. Some of them, such as refined grains, sweets, and soda pop should be avoided as much as possible for a lifetime of healthful eating and weight management.

Animal Proteins
Beef
    All fatty cuts (more toxins are stored in fat than muscle), which include: brisket, liver, liverwurst, rib eye steak, ribs
Pork in general, but especially avoid: bacon, honey-baked ham
Poultry
    Duck
    Goose
    Processed poultry products

Beverages
Alcohol: beer, liquor, wine
Anything with artificial flavors or sweeteners
Chocolate drinks/cocoa
Coffee
Diet sodas and all other sodas
Sports drinks
Fruit juice

Dairy
Ice cream
Milk

Processed cheese
Yogurt

Fats
Commercial salad dressings made with any of the oils listed below

Margarine
Polyunsaturated oils: canola, corn, peanut, safflower, sesame, soybean, sunflower

Fruit

Apple and applesauce
Apricot
Banana
Berries: blackberries, blueberries, boysenberries, gooseberries, loganberries, raspberries
Cherry
Date
Fig
Grapefruit
Grapes: green and red
Guava
Kiwifruit
Kumquat
Loquat
Lychee

Mango
Melons: cantaloupe, crenshaw, honeydew, watermelon
Nectarine
Orange
Papaya
Passion fruit
Peach
Pear
Persimmon
Pineapple
Plum
Pomegranate
Raisin
Rhubarb
Strawberry
Tangerine

Grains

Amaranth
Bagel
Biscuit
Bread
Bread stick
Breakfast pastry
Bun

Cereal
Cereal bar
Cracker
Doughnut
English muffin
Muffin
Oatmeal

Pancake
Pasta
Pizza dough
Quinoa
Roll

Spelt
Stuffing
Tortilla (corn and wheat)
Waffle
Wheat

Milk
Soy milk/dairy milk

Snack Foods
Cheese snacks
Chips: corn, potato, tortilla
Popcorn
Pretzels
Vegetable chips and snacks
Soy crisps and snacks

Sweets
Barbecue sauce with sweetener
Desserts: brownies, candy, cakes, cookies, frozen yogurt, gelatin, mousse, ice cream, pies, pudding, sorbet, whipped topping
Energy bars
Jams
Jellies
Ketchup
Sugar and sweeteners: all artificial sweeteners, brown sugar, brown rice syrup, honey, maple syrup, molasses, powdered sugar, white (refined and unrefined) sugar, fructose corn syrup

Vegetables
Corn
Jerusalem artichoke
Parsnip
Potatoes, all varieties, which include: Idaho, new white, red skinned

Squash: acorn, buttercup, butternut, spaghetti
Sweet potato
Yam
Yuca

JUICING FOR WEIGHT LOSS

Vegetable juice (not fruit juice) is recommended for The Coconut Diet. Vegetable juice offers an abundance of nutrients that feed the body superior nutrition. It is packed with appetite-suppressing soluble fiber and replete with vitamins and minerals, which help you start your day satisfied—and still able to peel off the pounds! If you follow the recommendations, you should not feel starved at any time on this diet. Fat cells respond to starvation by holding on to fat. The body's designed this way to keep human beings alive in times of famine.

When you skip breakfast or other meals, the brain sends a signal to your body that it's starving. This causes your body to store or hold on to fat for future use. Fresh vegetable juice in the morning provides your body with a host of nutrients and enzymes that supercharge your cells. It can help your brain function better all morning. Juice is known as a "live food," meaning it has not had its vitamins and enzymes destroyed by heat or processing, which means it's alive with nutrients! When your cells are well fed, you will have the energy to meet the day's demands.

For these reasons, though not mandatory, I recommend a glass of fresh vegetable juice each day of your 21 days of Phase I and throughout Phases II and III. You can take fresh juice to work in a thermos, or drink it before you leave home. It's fabulous in providing energizing nutrients that tell your body: you aren't hungry anymore!

You'll need a good juicer to make juicing an easy fit to your lifestyle. If you don't already have a good juicer, choose one that is easy to clean, is stainless steel, and has a good motor (½-hp). You can read more about the juicing at www.juicinginfo.com.

THE 1-DAY JUICE CLEANSE

You can try the 1-Day Vegetable Juice Cleanse for one, two, or all three weeks of Phase I. This is an all-liquid day that helps facilitate faster weight loss. Consider choosing a weekend day or any other day when you don't have to work outside your home. During that day you will drink only vegetable juices, vegetable broth, water, sparkling mineral water, and herbal or green teas. That's all. This day is a great boost to weight loss and will especially help you get rid of excess stored water and toxins. It also helps to rejuvenate the entire body.

The 1-Day Juice Cleanse Menu

Note: Recipes follow the day's menu.

Breakfast
Herbal or green tea with lemon juice or
Hot water with lemon and a dash of cayenne pepper and Morning Energy Cocktail or vegetable juice of choice

Mid-Morning
9:30 a.m. 8 ounces of water*
10:30 a.m. Herbal tea, green tea, or vegetable juice
11:30 a.m. 8 ounces of water

Lunch
V-8 juice or Spicy Tomato on Ice

Mid-Afternoon
1:30 p.m. 8 ounces water
2:30 p.m. 8 ounces water

*Sparkling mineral water may be substituted for water at any time. Add a squeeze of lemon or lime for added flavor, or a dash of unsweetened cranberry juice.

3:00 p.m. Herbal tea, green tea, warm vegetable broth, or vegetable juice

4:00 p.m. 8 ounces water

5:00 p.m. 8 ounces water

Dinner

8 to 10 ounces of vegetable juice of choice or

Cold Cucumber Avocado Soup

(You may also add a cup of warm vegetable broth.)

Low-Carb Vegetable Juice Recipes

Morning Energy Cocktail

If you think vegetable juice is going to be a taste challenge, try this recipe. It's not only delicious, it's loaded with antioxidants. This juice combo has about 17 carbs. It's a good carb investment considering it's replete with antioxidants, soluble fiber, enzymes, phytochemicals, minerals, and other nutrients.

Serves 1

1 cucumber, peeled if not organic
½ lemon, peeled
1 carrot, scrubbed
2 stalks celery
Handful parsley
1-inch piece ginger root

Cut the cucumber in half and push half the cucumber through the juicer. Follow with the lemon and carrot, then the other ingredients and end with the other half of the cucumber.

Stir and drink as soon as possible.

Nutritional breakdown per serving (based on 1 carrot): 155 calories (7% from fat); 1 g fat; 5 g protein; 17 g carbohydrate; >2 g dietary fiber; 0 mg cholesterol; 115 mg sodium.

Spicy Tomato on Ice

This is a refreshing drink especially in the afternoon, but good any time of day.

SERVES 1

1 vine-ripened tomato
1 cucumber, peeled if not organic
2 stalks celery
Dash of hot sauce
Ice cubes (optional)

Cut the tomato into chunks to fit your juicer and cut the cucumber in half, lengthwise.

Juice the tomato, cucumber, and celery.

Add a dash of hot sauce to taste and stir. Serve over ice.

Nutritional breakdown per serving: 39 calories (9.9% from fat); 1 g fat; 2 g protein; 9 g carbohydrate; >2 g dietary fiber; 0 mg cholesterol; 96 mg sodium.

Cold Cucumber Avocado Soup

This is a filling, satisfying cold soup.

SERVES 2

1½ cups fresh cucumber juice from 2 large cucumbers
¼ cup fresh lemon juice
1 tablespoon chopped green onion
1 tablespoon chopped red onion
1 tablespoon chopped fresh parsley
1 large ripe avocado, peeled and seeded
1 large or 2 medium garlic cloves, minced
3 sprigs fresh basil, chopped (optional)
1 teaspoon tamari or light soy sauce
1 to 2 teaspoons curry powder, or to taste

½ **teaspoon ground cumin**
Fresh basil, for garnish

Combine the juices and remaining ingredients in a blender and puree until smooth. If the soup is a bit too thick, add a little more cucumber juice or lemon juice.

Pour the soup into bowls and serve cold. Garnish with fresh basil or any other fresh herb of choice.

Nutritional breakdown per serving: 186 calories (68.9% from fat); 16 g fat; 3 g protein; 13 g carbohydrate; 4 g dietary fiber; 0 mg cholesterol; 182 mg sodium.

PREVENT GALLSTONES DURING WEIGHT LOSS

During weight loss, concentration of cholesterol in the bile actually increases, setting the stage for gallstones. Secretion of all bile components is reduced during weight loss, but secretion of bile acids decreases more than cholesterol. One function of bile acids is to keep cholesterol in solution. This setup greatly increases the risk of gallstone formation or acceleration.

Once weight is stabilized, bile acid output returns to normal and the cholesterol production remains low. The overall effect is an improvement in bile solubility with weight loss. For this reason, consider a liver/gallbladder cleanse during weight loss (see chapter 7, "Phase II: Cleansing"). In addition, you should follow the general guidelines for gallstone prevention.

General Guidelines for Gallstone Prevention

○ **Eat fiber-rich foods.** Research indicates that a fiber-depleted diet is one of the primary causes of gallstones. A diet low in fiber can lead to a reduction in bile acids produced in the liver and lower bile acid concentration in the

continued on next page

gallbladder. Eat lots of vegetables, flax seeds (ground), and a small amount of legumes.

O **Fish oils may be beneficial.** Animal studies have shown that the addition of fish oil inhibits gallstone formation. Cod liver oil is a good choice. Before you dismiss this idea as the worst possible thought, try a flavored cod liver oil. Flavored cod liver oil is not bad. And you can quickly chase it with lemon water or vegetable juice. It also does wonders for dry skin and is helpful for hypothyroid because it is rich in vitamin A. (People who have low thyroid seem to have challenges converting beta-carotene to vitamin A.)

O **Avoid coffee.** Coffee (even decaffeinated) causes gallbladder contractions.

O **Drink plenty of water.** Drink eight to ten 8-ounce glasses of water per day to maintain the water content of the bile.

O **Take vitamins C and E.** Animal studies have shown that deficiencies of vitamins E and C can cause gallstones. Vitamin C has shown positive effects on bile composition and has reduced gallstone formation.[5]

THE MENU PLAN

Delicious recipes and menu suggestions that utilize coconut oil provide great ideas for ways to incorporate coconut oil into your diet and recipe preparation, with ingredients that can be found in almost any grocery store. For the next three weeks you can use the guidelines that follow.

Basic Guidelines

Drink at least 8–10 glasses of water each day. The current recommendation from many holistic doctors is that you drink one quart of water for each 50 pounds of body weight. For example, if you weigh more than 100 pounds, you should be drinking more than eight glasses of water per day. Drinking adequate water will facilitate weight loss, and purified water is best. Sometimes we think we're hungry when we're actually thirsty. Drink a glass of water about 30 minutes before mealtime and you should not be as hungry and should actually eat less food.

Consume two to three tablespoons of coconut oil each day. You can cook with the oil, add it to Smoothies such as the Low-Carb Coconut Smoothie (page 177), or make it into Coconut Treats (page 211).

Design your Coconut Diet program to meet your particular needs. The 21-day menu plan and recipes are guidelines. You may pick and choose what fits your lifestyle. The important thing is that you avoid the carbohydrates and other foods that are listed on the foods to avoid list (beginning on page 128).

When eating out, say, "No bread, please." It helps a lot when dining in restaurants to tell the waitperson not to bring bread to the table. Those warm rolls and butter are often just too tempting when you're hungry and waiting for your meal. Order hamburgers without the bun and sandwiches without the bread.

I have started cooking more with virgin coconut oil. *Wow*—what a taste sensation! I thought it would be "icky" on eggs and in stir-fry; instead, I have found that it just enhances the flavor of foods. It's really not "coconutty." So if you haven't thought of cooking with virgin coconut oil, give it a try.

—*Kate*

DAY 1

Breakfast
Green or herbal tea with a slice of lemon
6 to 8 ounces vegetable juice, preferably fresh
Basic Scrambled Eggs (page 154)

1 slice turkey bacon
2 slices fresh tomato sprinkled with fresh or dried herbs of choice

Mid-Morning Break
Green or herbal tea with lemon
12 raw or toasted almonds

Lunch
Crispy Coconut Chicken Salad (page 162)

Mid-Afternoon Snack
Sparkling mineral water with a slice of lemon
1 stalk celery stuffed with soft goat cheese; cut into 6 pieces

Dinner
Chicken with Citrus-Garlic-Ginger Sauce (page 183)
Steamed spinach (drizzle some of the Citrus-Garlic-Ginger Sauce
    over the spinach; it's delicious)
Mixed green salad with vinaigrette (see pages 172–176)
Coconut Treat (page 211)

DAY 2

Breakfast
Green or herbal tea with lemon
6 to 8 ounces vegetable juice, preferably fresh
Veggie Scramble (page 155)
1 slice turkey or beef bacon

Mid-Morning Break
Green or herbal tea
Celery sticks stuffed with soft goat cheese, cut into 6 pieces

Lunch
Chicken Salad Stuffed Tomato (page 164)

Mid-Afternoon Snack
Herbal tea (iced or hot) with a slice of lemon
Coconut Treat (page 211)

Dinner
Grilled Lamb Salad with Minted Balsamic Dressing (page 165)
Cup of soup such as Tomato-Basil (page 288)

DAY 3

Breakfast
Green or herbal tea with lemon
Sun-dried tomato and feta Cheese Omelet (page 157)
    (Start with the Basic Cheese Omelet, page 157, and add feta and
chopped sun-dried tomatoes.)

Mid-Morning Break
6 to 8 ounces vegetable juice, preferably fresh
1 celery stalk stuffed with soft goat cheese, cut into six pieces

Lunch
Cup of Gazpacho soup (page 177)
Healthy Hamburger (page 185)

Mid-Afternoon Snack
Sparkling mineral water with a slice of lime
2 slices deli turkey or roast beef

Dinner
Marinated steak (page 199)
Steamed snow peas
Mixed green salad with cucumber, tomato, green onions, and grated
    carrot with vinaigrette (pages 172–176)

DAY 4

Breakfast
Green or herbal tea with lemon
Low-Carb Coconut Smoothie (page 153)

Mid-Morning Break
1 hard-boiled egg
6 to 8 ounces vegetable juice, preferably fresh

Lunch
Tasty Greens Sauté (page 180) with diced chicken

Mid-Afternoon Snack
3 to 4 sardines, packed in mustard sauce

Dinner
Chicken Breasts in Chunky Tomato-Vegetable Sauce (page 202)
Steamed vegetables of choice
Sliced tomatoes with fresh or dried herbs of choice and a drizzle of
    balsamic vinegar and extra-virgin olive oil

DAY 5

Breakfast
Green or herbal tea with lemon
6 to 8 ounces vegetable juice, preferably fresh
Vegetable Quiche On-the-Go (page 161)

Mid-Morning Break
Herbal tea (iced or hot)
6 macadamia nuts

Lunch
Napa Cabbage-Carrot Salad (page 167)
Cup of low-carb soup

Mid-Afternoon Snack
Sparkling mineral water with a slice of lemon
2 to 3 slices deli turkey

Dinner
Fish in Fennel Sauce (page 186)
Steamed green beans and sliced onions
Crisp garden salad with Lemon Vinaigrette (page 163)

DAY 6

Breakfast
Green or herbal tea with lemon
6 to 8 ounces vegetable juice, preferably fresh
Basic Frittata (page 158)

Mid-Morning Break
1 stalk celery stuffed with soft goat cheese, cut into six pieces

Lunch
Spinach salad with pistachio nuts, ½ avocado, cherry tomatoes, and
    crumbled feta cheese with Lemon Vinaigrette (page 163)
Cup of Gazpacho soup (page 177)

Mid-Afternoon Snack
Coconut Treat (page 211)

Dinner
Golden Chicken (page 188)
Steamed cauliflower with a little butter and seasoning (or you can
    whip cauliflower and make mock mashed potatoes)
Crispy green salad with olive oil and vinegar dressing or Basic
    Vinaigrette (page 172)

DAY 7

Breakfast
Green or herbal tea with lemon
Eggs Benedict on Turkey Ham (page 159)

Mid-Morning Break
Vegetable sticks with herbed mayonnaise (see Virgin Coconut Oil
    Mayonnaise on page 208 and add your favorite chopped herbs)

Lunch
Steamed Vegetable Salad (page 169)
1 piece Golden Chicken left over from the day before

Mid-Afternoon Snack
6 to 8 ounces vegetable juice, preferably fresh

Dinner
Chicken in Coconut Milk with Lime Leaves (page 189)
Steamed asparagus or spinach (drizzle some of the coconut milk
    sauce over the vegetables)
Sliced cucumber and onion with rice vinegar on crispy greens

DAY 8

Breakfast
Green or herbal tea with lemon
6 to 8 ounces vegetable juice, preferably fresh
Basic Cheese Omelet, with Cheddar (page 157)

Mid-Morning Break
2 Turkey Roll-Ups (page 210)

Lunch
Beet-Sauerkraut Salad (page 170)
Cup of low-carb soup

Mid-Afternoon Snack
Sparkling mineral water with a slice of lemon or lime
12 raw or toasted almonds

Dinner
Turkey Stew (page 179)
Spinach salad with Lemon-Chive Vinaigrette (page 174)

DAY 9

Breakfast
Green or herbal tea with lemon
Vegetable Quiche On-the-Go (page 161)
1 to 2 slices turkey or beef bacon

Mid-Morning Break
6 to 8 ounces vegetable juice, preferably fresh
12 raw or toasted almonds

Lunch
Curried Chicken Salad (page 171)

Mid-Afternoon Snack
Sparkling mineral water with a slice of lemon
Vegetable sticks

Dinner
Stuffed Rainbow Trout Filets (page 190)
Steamed green beans
Crispy green salad with Tarragon Vinaigrette (page 175)

DAY 10

Breakfast
Green or herbal tea with lemon
Low-Carb Coconut Smoothie (page 153)

Mid-Morning Break
6 to 8 ounces vegetable juice, preferably fresh
1 hard-boiled egg

Lunch
Caesar salad with grilled chicken

Mid-Afternoon Snack
6 pecan halves
Sparkling mineral water with a slice of lemon

Dinner
Lamb and Eggplant Casserole (page 192)
Crispy salad with Basic Vinaigrette (page 172)

DAY 11

Breakfast
Green or herbal tea with lemon
Asian Scramble (page 156)

Mid-Morning Break
6 to 8 ounces vegetable juice, preferably fresh
12 raw or toasted almonds

Lunch
Thai Chicken Soup with Coconut and Galanga (page 178)

Mid-Afternoon Snack
Sparkling mineral water with a slice of lemon
1 stalk celery stuffed with soft goat cheese, cut into six pieces

Dinner
Salmon Steaks with Vegetables (page 194)
Crispy green salad with Mustard Vinaigrette (page 175)

DAY 12

Breakfast
Green or herbal tea with lemon
6 to 8 ounces fresh vegetable juice
Basic Scrambled Eggs (page 154)

Mid-Morning Break
6 to 8 ounces vegetable juice, preferably fresh
12 raw or toasted almonds

Lunch
Cup of low-carb soup
Tomato-mozzarella salad with fresh basil and a drizzle of balsamic
    vinegar and extra-virgin olive oil

Mid-Afternoon Snack
Sparkling mineral water with a slice of lemon or lime
2 thin slices turkey breast

Dinner
Super-Speedy Supper (page 195)
Crispy green salad with Basic Vinaigrette (page 172)

DAY 13

Breakfast
Green or herbal tea with lemon
6 to 8 ounces vegetable juice, preferably fresh
1 poached egg
2 strips turkey or beef bacon

Mid-Morning Break
Herbal or green tea
6 to 12 raw or toasted almonds

Lunch
Bowl of Tomato Basil Soup (page 288)
Green salad with Garlic Vinaigrette (page 173)

Mid-Afternoon Snack
Sparkling mineral water with a slice of lemon
Coconut Treat (page 211)

Dinner
Lemon Tarragon Fish (page 196)
Wild rice (¼ cup per serving)
Steamed asparagus and globe artichokes
Sliced tomatoes sprinkled with herbs of choice and a drizzle of
    balsamic vinegar and extra-virgin olive oil

DAY 14

Breakfast
Green or herbal tea with lemon
6 to 8 ounces fresh vegetable juice
Basic Cheese Omelet (page 157)
1 slice turkey bacon

Mid-Morning Break
Green or herbal tea with lemon
6 macadamia nuts

Lunch
Chef salad with Basic Vinaigrette (page 172) or dressing of
    choice

Mid-Afternoon Snack
Sparkling mineral water with lemon slices
3 radishes and 4 green olives

Dinner
Stuffed Beef Rolls (page 197)
Steamed vegetable medley
Crispy garden salad with Caper and Egg Vinaigrette (page 173)

DAY 15

Breakfast
Green or herbal tea with lemon
6 to 8 ounces fresh vegetable juice
Basic Frittata (page 158)

Mid-Morning Break
Green or herbal tea with lemon
6 pecan halves

Lunch
Bowl of Chili (page 184)
Green salad with Basic Vinaigrette (page 172)

Mid-Afternoon Snack
Sparkling mineral water with lemon slices
2 Beef Roll-Ups (page 210)

Dinner
Baked Lemon Chicken Thighs (page 198)
Steamed broccoli and cauliflower
Caesar salad

DAY 16

Breakfast
Green or herbal tea with lemon
Low-Carb Coconut Smoothie (page 153)

Mid-Morning Break
6 to 8 ounces of vegetable juice, preferably fresh
1 hard-boiled egg

Lunch
Healthy Hamburger (page 185)
Crispy green salad with Mustard Vinaigrette (page 175)

Mid-Afternoon Snack
Sparkling mineral water with a slice of lemon
12 raw or toasted almonds

Dinner
Marinated Steak (page 199)
Steamed vegetable medley
Crispy garden salad with Garlic Vinaigrette (page 173)

DAY 17

Breakfast
Green or herbal tea with lemon
6 to 8 ounces vegetable juice, preferably fresh
Basic Scrambled Eggs (page 154)
1 slice of turkey or beef bacon

Mid-Morning Break
Green or herbal tea with lemon
Slice of goat cheese

Lunch
Half avocado stuffed with tuna salad
Cup of Gazpacho soup (page 177)

Mid-Afternoon Snack
Sparkling mineral water with a slice of lemon
Veggie sticks

Dinner
Turkey in Coconut Milk (page 200)
Wild rice
A salad of finely sliced cucumbers, celery, and lettuce with Lemon-
Chive Vinaigrette (page 174)

DAY 18

Breakfast
Green or herbal tea with lemon
6 to 8 ounces vegetable juice, preferably fresh
Scrambled eggs with spinach and feta cheese
1 slice turkey or beef bacon

Mid-Morning Break
Green or herbal tea with lemon
6 to 10 raw or toasted almonds

Lunch
Turkey Cobb salad: lettuce, turkey, hard-boiled egg, crumbled
bacon, cherry tomatoes with mustard-mayonnaise dressing

Mid-Afternoon Snack
Sparkling mineral water with a slice of lemon or lime
A celery stick stuffed with soft goat cheese, cut into 6 pieces

Dinner
Baked Drumsticks with Spicy Eggplant (page 201)
Spinach salad with your favorite vinaigrette (pages 172–176)
Coconut Treat (page 211)

DAY 19

Breakfast
Green or herbal tea with lemon
6 to 8 ounces vegetable juice, preferably fresh
Unbelievable Baked Eggs (page 162)
1 slice of turkey or beef bacon

Mid-Morning Break
Green or herbal tea with lemon
2 dozen raw sunflower seeds

Lunch
Grilled salmon Caesar salad

Mid-Afternoon Snack
Sparkling mineral water with a slice of lemon or lime
Celery stuffed with 1 teaspoon of macadamia nut butter

Dinner
Broiled fish with Asian Pesto (page 209)
Artichokes with Hollandaise Sauce (page 181)
Crispy garden salad with your favorite vinaigrette
   (pages 172–176)

DAY 20

Breakfast
Green or herbal tea with lemon
6 to 8 ounces vegetable juice, preferably fresh
South-of-the-Border Scrambled Eggs (page 154)

Mid-Morning Break
Green or herbal tea with lemon

Lunch
2 Beef Roll-Ups (page 210) with garden salad

Mid-Afternoon Snack
Sparkling mineral water with a slice of lemon or lime
2 dozen toasted pumpkin seeds

Dinner
Sautéed Chicken Breasts with Pico de Gallo (page 203)
Steamed green beans
Crispy green salad with Lemon–Chive Vinaigrette (page 174)

DAY 21

Breakfast
Green or herbal tea with lemon
6 to 8 ounces vegetable juice, preferably fresh
Eggs Benedict Florentine (page 160)

Mid-Morning Break
Green or herbal tea with lemon
6 to 10 raw or toasted almonds

Lunch
Grilled salmon Caesar salad

Mid-Afternoon Snack
Sparkling mineral water with a slice of lemon or lime
Veggie sticks

Dinner
Sautéed Chicken Breasts with Tomato Sauce (page 205)
Crispy garden salad with Garlic Vinaigrette (page 173)

Daily Food Log and Planner

Virgin coconut oil _____ (minimum 2–3 tablespoons per day)

Water _____ minimum eight 8-ounce glasses per day

Herbal tea   Green tea

Food List

_____ Legumes   _____ Fat

Meat/Fish/Poultry   Fruit

_____ Vegetables   _____ Other

Vitamin/Mineral supplements

Meal Planner

Breakfast

_____

_____

Mid-Morning Break

_____

Lunch

_____

_____

Mid-Afternoon Snack

_____

Dinner

_____

_____

BREAKFAST RECIPES

Low-Carb Coconut Smoothie

This is a quick breakfast you can drink on the go!

SERVES 2

1 cup Coconut Milk (page 206) or 1 (13.5-ounce) can coconut
milk or 1 cup Almond Milk (page 207)*
1 to 2 tablespoons protein powder (goat protein, whey, or rice
protein)
1 tablespoon virgin coconut oil
1 tablespoon ground flax seeds
1 teaspoon pure vanilla extract
¼ teaspoon almond extract
¼ teaspoon stevia powder or equivalent sweetener
8 to 10 ice cubes

Place all ingredients except ice in a blender and process at high
speed until well combined.

Add ice after the coconut oil is blended so that it won't clump.
Use more or less ice, depending on cold preference.

*A 13.5-ounce can of coconut milk yields 7 grams of carbs or 3.5
grams per serving. Packaged almond milk yields about 8 grams of
carbs per cup.

Nutritional breakdown per serving: 310 calories (85.8% from fat); 32 g fat; 4 g protein; 8 g carbohydrate; 4 g dietary fiber; 0 mg cholesterol; 27 mg sodium.

Basic Scrambled Eggs

This makes a nice quick breakfast on a busy morning.

SERVES 2

4 large eggs
2 tablespoons heavy cream or milk of choice (plain, almond, or rice)
Black pepper, freshly ground
2 tablespoons virgin coconut oil

In a medium bowl, whisk eggs, cream, and black pepper. Set aside. In a medium-size nonstick skillet, melt coconut oil over medium-high heat. When oil is hot and bubbly, add eggs to pan. Reduce heat to medium. Gently stir egg mixture around with a wooden spoon, stirring until eggs are soft, creamy, and cooked to your liking. Serve immediately.

Nutritional breakdown per serving: 189 calories (71% from fat); 15 g fat; 11 g protein; 2 g carbohydrate; 0 g dietary fiber; 394 mg cholesterol; 116 mg sodium.

South-of-the-Border Scrambled Eggs

Start with the Basic Scrambled Eggs (above) and add the following ingredients:

SERVES 2

1 vine-ripened tomato, peeled, seeded, and chopped
1 tablespoon chopped green pepper
1 tablespoon chopped parsley
2 tablespoons chopped chives

In a medium bowl, beat the eggs and cream. Add tomato, green pepper, and parsley; stir well to combine.

Melt coconut oil in a medium-size heavy skillet. When oil is shimmering (shining with flickering light), pour in egg mixture; cook, stirring frequently with spatula, until just done. Do not overcook or eggs will be rubbery. Sprinkle with chives and serve immediately.

Nutritional breakdown per serving: 187 calories (63.6% from fat); 13 g fat; 12 g protein; 5 g carbohydrate; 1 g dietary fiber; 387 mg cholesterol; 123 mg sodium.

Veggie Scramble

This is one way to get more vegetables in your diet!

Serves 2

1 tablespoon virgin coconut oil
2 tablespoons zucchini, chopped
1 tablespoon onion, minced
2 cherry tomatoes, quartered
4 large eggs
1 tablespoon milk, cream, or plain almond milk
Sea salt or Celtic salt
Black pepper, freshly ground

In a small pan, melt the coconut oil. Add the zucchini and onions and sauté until tender.

Next, add the cherry tomatoes, stir and sauté for 2 minutes.

While the vegetables are sautéing, beat the eggs with milk or cream in a small bowl. Add salt and pepper, to taste.

Pour eggs into the pan and scramble lightly; overcooking eggs will cause them to turn rubbery.

Nutritional breakdown per serving: 147 calories (58.9% from fat); 10 g fat; 12 g protein; 3 g carbohydrate; trace dietary fiber; 375 mg cholesterol; 117 mg sodium.

Asian Scramble

A delicious variation on scrambled eggs!

SERVES 2

4 large eggs
2 tablespoons heavy cream or milk of choice (plain, almond, or rice)
Black pepper, freshly ground
2 tablespoons virgin coconut oil
2 tablespoons scallions, minced
2 tablespoons fresh cilantro, minced
1 teaspoon fresh ginger, peeled and finely minced
¼ cup celery, thinly sliced
1 cup fresh mushrooms, sliced
2 teaspoons low-sodium soy sauce

In a medium bowl, whisk eggs, cream, and black pepper. Set aside.

In a medium-size skillet, heat oil over medium-high heat. When oil is hot and bubbly, add scallions, cilantro, ginger, celery, and mushrooms, and sauté about 5 minutes. Drain excess liquid from pan.

Add egg mixture and gently stir eggs around with a wooden spoon, until eggs are soft, creamy, and cooked to your liking. Serve immediately.

Nutritional breakdown per serving: 443 calories (61.6% calories from fat); 30 g fat; 36 g protein; 6 g carbohydrate; 1 g dietary fiber; 574 mg cholesterol; 508 mg sodium.

Basic Cheese Omelet

Start with this basic omelet and you can add fillings of your choice.

SERVES 2

4 large eggs
2 tablespoons heavy cream or milk of choice (plain, almond, or rice)
Black pepper, freshly ground
2 tablespoons virgin coconut oil
¼ cup cheddar cheese or cheese of choice, grated or crumbled

In a medium bowl, whisk eggs, cream, and black pepper. Set aside.

In a medium-size nonstick skillet, melt 2 tablespoons coconut oil over medium-high heat. When oil is hot and bubbly, add egg mixture, reduce heat to medium and cook, lifting edges to allow uncooked egg to seep underneath.

When bottom layer of egg mixture is cooked but top is still moist, sprinkle grated or crumbled cheese over one side of omelet. Gently fold omelet in half. Cook half a minute longer.

Slide omelet onto plate and serve immediately.

Nutritional breakdown per serving: 357 calories (81.7% from fat); 33 g fat; 15 g protein; 2 g carbohydrate; 0 g dietary fiber; 409 mg cholesterol; 204 mg sodium.

Basic Frittata

On the weekend, or any day you have the time, a frittata is a nice change from the usual fare. You can add any filling you like to this basic recipe. A frittata also makes a nice entrée for dinner.

SERVES 2

4 large eggs
2 tablespoons heavy cream or milk of choice (plain, almond or rice)
2 teaspoons fresh herbs such as parsley, basil, thyme, or oregano, minced
Black pepper, freshly ground
Dash cayenne pepper
2 tablespoons virgin coconut oil
½ cup mozzarella cheese, grated

Preheat broiler.

In a medium bowl, whisk eggs, cream, fresh herbs, black pepper, and cayenne pepper. Set aside.

In a medium-size oven-proof skillet, melt coconut oil over medium-high heat. When oil is hot and bubbly, add egg mixture. As eggs cook, lift edges to allow uncooked egg mixture to seep underneath. When bottom is set but top is still moist, spread cheese over eggs and place under broiler.

Broil 1 to 2 minutes, checking frequently, until top is golden and puffed up.

Nutritional breakdown per serving: 678 calories (75.5% from fat); 57 g fat; 37 g protein; 5 g carbohydrate; trace dietary fiber; 500 mg cholesterol; 609 mg sodium.

Eggs Benedict with Turkey Ham

Serve with Classic Blender Hollandaise Sauce (page 160) and without the English muffin.

SERVES 4

**1 tablespoon virgin coconut oil
4 slices turkey ham, nitrate free
Water
1 tablespoon white vinegar
8 large eggs**

In a skillet, heat virgin coconut oil until shimmering. Cook turkey ham over low heat until lightly crisped. Remove from pan and blot with paper towels.

In a deep skillet, bring 2 inches of water and vinegar to a boil over high heat. Reduce heat to a simmer.

Crack eggs, one at a time, into a small bowl and tip gently into simmering water. Repeat with all eggs. Cover skillet and cook: 3 minutes for soft yolks, 5 minutes for firmer yolks.

Using a slotted spoon, remove eggs from water and drain thoroughly.

Top each slice of turkey ham with a poached egg. Follow with Classic Blender Hollandaise sauce (page 160).

Nutritional breakdown per serving: 614 (70.6% from fat); 49 g fat; 22 g protein; 23 g carbohydrate; 9 g dietary fiber; 658 mg cholesterol; 893 mg sodium.

Classic Blender Hollandaise Sauce

This hollandaise sauce is very easy to make.

MAKES 6 OUNCES: 12 SERVINGS

3 large egg yolks, whole
2 tablespoons fresh lemon juice
1 dash cayenne pepper
4 ounces unsalted butter, melted and bubbling hot

In a blender, combine egg yolks, lemon juice, and cayenne pepper and blend on high for 3 seconds.

Remove lid and, with motor running, slowly pour hot butter in a steady stream over egg mixture. When butter is all poured in, blend an additional 5 seconds. Taste and adjust seasonings.

Serve immediately or keep sauce warm by placing blender in a bowl of warm water.

Nutritional breakdown per serving: 83 calories (94.8% from fat); 9 g fat; 1 g protein; trace carbohydrate; trace dietary fiber; 74 mg cholesterol; 3 mg sodium.

Eggs Benedict Florentine or Eggs Benedict Oscar

Start with the Eggs Benedict on Turkey Ham (page 159) and substitute steamed spinach or 4 crab cakes as the bed for the poached eggs. Either steam a pound of fresh spinach or cook 1 (10-ounce) package frozen spinach or 4 pre-made crab cakes. Drain and spoon a couple of heaping tablespoons of spinach on a plate and pat or place on a crab cake to form a bed for each poached egg. Spoon the Classic Blender Hollandaise Sauce (above) over top and serve immediately.

Vegetable Quiche On-the-Go

Make these quiche cups ahead on the weekend, and you can warm them up on busy weekdays. They can also be frozen and reheated. You may add any vegetables of your liking or chopped turkey or crumbled beef or turkey bacon.

SERVES 6

1 (10-ounce) package frozen chopped spinach, thawed
2 tablespoons virgin coconut oil
¼ cup diced onions
¼ cup chopped sun-dried tomatoes or chopped bell pepper
3 eggs, beaten
¾ cup grated Swiss cheese
½ cup cream
Sea salt or Celtic salt and pepper, to taste

Cook spinach according to directions; drain excess liquid.

Line a 12-cup muffin pan with foil baking cups. Melt 1 tablespoon of coconut oil and brush each cup with oil.

Melt the other tablespoon of coconut oil in a small sauté pan and sauté onions and sun-dried tomatoes or bell pepper for about 5 minutes on medium-low heat, or until tender.

While vegetables are sautéing, beat the eggs in a medium-size bowl. Add the cheese and cream and mix until combined. Add the spinach, onion, sun-dried tomatoes or bell pepper, and salt and pepper to taste. Stir until well combined.

Divide the mixture evenly among the cups and bake at 350 degrees F for 20 minutes, or until knife inserted in the center comes out clean.

Nutritional breakdown per serving: 153 calories (65.5% from fat); 11 g fat; 9 g protein; 5 g carbohydrate; 2 g dietary fiber; 124 mg cholesterol; 154 mg sodium.

Unbelievable Baked Eggs

My Aunt Millie made these eggs for me nearly every time I visited for a weekend. They were one of her favorites—and mine. They make a very easy breakfast. You simply put the eggs in the oven. And since you don't have to watch them, you can concentrate on other morning activities.

SERVES 1

1–2 teaspoons virgin coconut oil
1 to 2 eggs
1 to 2 tablespoons cream
Sea salt or Celtic salt and pepper, to taste

Preheat oven to 350 degrees F.

Melt coconut oil in ramekin or any individual baking dish. Crack one or two eggs into ramekin, top with cream and salt and pepper.

Bake for 15 minutes, or until yolk reaches desired firmness. If you like the yolk a little firmer, bake another 10 minutes.

Nutritional breakdown per serving: 86 calories (70.1% from fat); 7 g fat; 6 g protein; 1 carbohydrate; 0 g dietary fiber; 191 mg cholesterol; 292 mg sodium.

SALADS

Crispy Coconut Chicken Salad

This is a very delicious salad and it's easy to make.

SERVES 2

2 boneless, skinless chicken breasts
¼ cup unsweetened, finely shredded coconut
¼ cup ground flax seeds

1 egg, beaten
2 tablespoons virgin coconut oil
4 cups mixed greens, with vinaigrette

Rinse the chicken and pat dry; cut into strips, and set aside.

Mix shredded coconut and ground flax seeds together on a dinner plate.

In a small bowl, beat the egg, and dip the chicken strips in the beaten egg, then roll each chicken strip in the coconut-flax mixture.

Melt coconut oil in a medium-size frying pan.

Place chicken strips in hot oil; they should sizzle when placed in the pan. Sauté over medium heat until crispy on the outside. Turn after about 2 minutes and brown the other side of each chicken strip for another 2 minutes, or until completely opaque in the center. When done, remove chicken strips from pan and cool on paper towels.

Serve over a bed of mixed greens with Lemon Vinaigrette (below) or your favorite dressing.

Nutritional breakdown per serving: 340 calories (23% from fat); 9 g fat; 58 g protein; 6 g carbohydrate; 4 g dietary fiber; 237 mg cholesterol; 181 mg sodium.

Lemon Vinaigrette

Makes about 6 ounces: 4 servings

3 tablespoons fresh lemon juice
1 tablespoon (or equivalent) healthy, low-carb sweetener
2 tablespoons finely minced red onion
½ teaspoon lemon zest
¼ teaspoon sea salt or Celtic salt
¼ cup extra virgin olive oil

In a small bowl, whisk together all the dressing ingredients except the oil.

Slowly drizzle in the oil, holding it several inches above the bowl and pouring in a thin, steady stream, while whisking vigorously until the mixture thickens.

Nutritional breakdown per serving: 13 calories (15.9% from fat); 2 g fat; trace g protein; 3 g carbohydrate; trace g dietary fiber; 0 mg cholesterol; 6 mg sodium.

Chicken Salad Stuffed Tomato

This is a nice way to use leftover chicken from the evening before. Or to make sure you have enough chicken for lunch, just cook a little extra the night before.

SERVES 1

1 medium to large fresh tomato
½ cup chopped chicken (tuna can be substituted)
¼ cup Virgin Coconut Oil Mayonnaise (page 208) or mayonnaise of choice
¼ cup chopped celery
1 tablespoon slivered almonds
Salt and pepper, to taste

Cut about one-quarter of the top off the tomato. With a spoon, scoop out the flesh.

In a small bowl, combine the chicken, mayonnaise, celery, almonds, and salt and pepper, to taste.

Fill the tomato with the chicken salad.

Nutritional breakdown per serving: 268 calories (61.2% from fat); 19 g fat; 18 g protein; 9 g carbohydrate; 2 g dietary fiber; 78 mg cholesterol; 98 mg sodium.

Grilled Lamb Salad with Minted Balsamic Dressing

This is a delicious main-course salad that makes a great lunch or dinner entrée.

SERVES 4

Mint Marinade

¼ light soy sauce
1 tablespoon raspberry vinegar
1 tablespoon extra-virgin coconut oil (melted to liquid)
1 tablespoon chopped fresh mint or 1 teaspoon dried
1 teaspoon (or equivalent) low-carb healthy sweetener
¼ teaspoon freshly ground black pepper

Nutritional breakdown per serving: 14 calories (15.1% from fat); 2 g fat; 1 g protein; 2 g carbohydrate; trace g dietary fiber; 0 mg cholesterol; 602 mg sodium.

Minted Balsamic Dressing

¼ cup balsamic vinegar
1 tablespoon Dijon mustard
1 teaspoon (or equivalent) low-carb healthy sweetener
⅓ cup virgin coconut oil (melted) or extra-virgin olive oil
¼ teaspoon freshly ground black pepper
1 clove garlic, minced
1 tablespoon chopped fresh mint

Nutritional breakdown per serving: 34 calories (33.9% from fat); 2 g fat; 1 g protein; 6 g carbohydrate; 1 g dietary fiber; 0 mg cholesterol; 189 mg sodium.

Grilled Lamb Salad

This salad is a little extra work, but it's worth it!

½ pound lamb top round cut into steak, pounded and sliced
   against the grain* (or use leftover lamb from a previous meal,
   cut into strips)
4 skewers, if using outdoor grill
2 cups romaine lettuce, washed, dried, and torn into bite-size
   pieces
2 cups baby spring greens (mesclun)
½ cup chopped green onions
10 cherry tomatoes, halved or quartered
¼ cup toasted pine nuts**

To make the marinade, combine all ingredients in a medium bowl and mix well. Place the sliced lamb in the marinade, cover, and refrigerate for 1 to 4 hours.

To make the dressing, combine the vinegar, mustard, and sweetener. Drizzle in the oil slowly. (Tip: Hold the oil several inches above the bowl and pour a very thin stream of oil in the bowl, a little bit at a time, while whisking or stirring vigorously, to create a thicker, creamier dressing.) Add the pepper, garlic, and mint, and stir until well blended.

Prepare the grill or electric grilling machine.

If using a charcoal grill, thread the lamb onto skewers. Oil the grid and place it above the coals. Place the lamb skewers on the grid and cook for 2 minutes, baste, and turn. Cook for another 2 minutes for medium rare.

If using an electric grilling machine, place the lamb strips on the hot grill. Drizzle a bit of the marinade over the top and cook for 1 minute and 15 seconds for medium rare.

To assemble the salad, in a large bowl combine the leafy greens, green onions, and tomatoes; toss and mix. Divide evenly among 4 plates. Top each salad with grilled lamb strips and spoon the dressing over top. Sprinkle with toasted pine nuts, if using, and serve.

*To help slice meat more thinly, place it in the freezer for 20 to 30 minutes first. For easy-to-chew meat, always slice it against the grain.

**To toast nuts, place them on a baking sheet with a raised edge and bake at 250 degrees F for 25 to 30 minutes, or until they are golden. Watch closely to avoid burning them. Remove the nuts from the oven and set aside to cool; they will become crunchier and more flavorful as they cool.

Nutritional breakdown per serving: 184 calories (67.8% from fat); 14 g fat; 5 g protein; 5 g carbohydrate; 2 g dietary fiber; 31 mg cholesterol; 33 mg sodium.

Napa Cabbage-Carrot Salad

This is a beautiful salad filled with lots of color, which means plenty of antioxidants.

SERVES 2 TO 4 AS A SNACK OR LIGHT MEAL, OR IN COMBINATION
WITH A SOUP, IT'S QUITE A FILLING MEAL

2 cups raw grated carrots
2 cups finely shredded napa cabbage
2 stalks celery, sliced
1 green pepper, sliced
1 yellow pepper, sliced
1 sweet onion, sliced
½ cup green olives, sliced
1 cup chopped cilantro
1 cup coarsely shredded coconut
2 to 3 tablespoons Simple Olive Oil Mayonnaise (page 168) or
Virgin Coconut Oil Mayonnaise (page 208)

Grate the carrots on the coarse side of the grater.
Shred the cabbage finely, using the top end where the leaves are curly and tender.

Finely slice the celery, peppers, and onion and mix with the cabbage and carrots.

Add the olives, chopped cilantro, coconut, and mayonnaise.

Nutritional breakdown per serving: 198 calories (37% from fat); 9 g fat; 5 g protein; 29 g carbohydrate; 7 g fiber; 0 mg cholesterol; 260 mg sodium.

Simple Olive Oil Mayonnaise

It is extremely important to start with all ingredients at room temperature.

MAKES ABOUT 1 CUP: ABOUT 8 SERVINGS

1 raw free-range egg
1 teaspoon Dijon mustard
1 teaspoon fresh lemon juice
1 cup extra-virgin olive oil (or combination of ½ olive oil and
    ½ coconut oil)

Using a blender or food processor, put in the raw egg, mustard, and lemon juice.

Start the motor and add the oil in a thin but steady stream until the mixture is quite thick. The sound in the motor will be an indication of this. If the mixture won't get thick add some more oil.

Variation: Add a handful of fresh herbs at the start, which will give the mayonnaise a delightful color as well as a different taste. Also, to give the mayonnaise more "zing," add a small anchovy filet, or some capers. For even more flavor, add feta cheese.

Nutritional breakdown per serving (based on 16 servings): 248 calories (79% from fat); 28 g fat; 8 g protein; trace carbohydrate; trace dietary fiber; 23 mg cholesterol; 15 mg sodium.

Steamed Vegetable Salad

Not all salads need to be crispy and raw. This steamed vegetable salad is a nice change from the typical garden variety. With a piece or two of Golden Chicken (page 188) or a hard-boiled egg, this salad makes a very satisfying meal. If need be, precede it with a low-carb soup.

SERVES 4 TO 6

2 cups yellow string beans
2 cups broccoli florets
2 cups cauliflower florets
½ teaspoon sea salt or Celtic salt
1 cup red peppers, sliced
½ cup finely sliced purple onions
1 cup finely sliced radishes
¼ cup extra virgin olive oil
¼ cup unpasteurized apple cider vinegar
½ cup finely chopped fresh dill

The string beans should go in the steamer first, since they will take a little longer to cook than the other vegetables.

Break up the broccoli and cauliflower into florets and add to the steamer, sprinkle with the sea salt. Don't overcook the vegetables.

When the broccoli is done, it will turn a vivid green color. Remove it and the cauliflower and put them into a salad bowl.

Test the beans to see if they are cooked; remove when done.

While the vegetables are steaming, cut some red peppers into strips. If you find cooked peppers easier to digest than raw ones, then put them in the steamer as well.

Next, slice the onions and radishes very finely.

Combine all the cooked and raw vegetables.

Add some of the oil and vinegar as dressing (apply lightly, you don't want to end up with soggy vegetables) and then add some finely chopped dill.

Variation: Sauerkraut makes a lovely addition to this salad, providing some zing. It's also an excellent way to get more enzymes into your diet. If adding sauerkraut, reduce or omit the apple cider vinegar.

Nutritional breakdown per serving: 67 calories (15% from fat); 1 g fat; 3 g protein; 13 g carbohydrate; 4 g fiber; 59 mg calcium; 1 mg iron; 0 mg cholesterol; 40 mg sodium.

Beet-Sauerkraut Salad

Boiled eggs, pickled herring, leftover roast beef, lamb, or steak are all good accompaniments to this salad.

SERVES 2 TO 4

2 cups fresh raw beets, grated*
2 cups sauerkraut**
2 stalks celery, sliced
1 green pepper, sliced
1 sweet onion, sliced
1 cup finely chopped iceberg lettuce
1 teaspoon caraway seeds
¼ cup extra virgin olive oil
1 cup finely chopped fresh dill

Cut the leaves and stalks off the beets and reserve for another dish or for fresh vegetable juice.

Peel the beets and grate them on the coarse side of the grater and add sauerkraut.

Finely slice the celery, pepper, onion, and lettuce and mix with the beets and sauerkraut. You may want to chop the sauerkraut if the strands are particularly long.

Add the caraway seeds, the oil, and the dill and mix well.

*Once they are grated, raw beets will not last more than two days in the fridge. Use them up while they are very fresh and crunchy.

**When buying sauerkraut, check the label carefully. It should contain only cabbage and salt, nothing else. Buy it in glass jars rather than cans.

Nutritional breakdown per serving: 197 calories (55% from fat); 14 g fat; 3 g protein; 17 g carbohydrate; 7 g fiber; 74 mg calcium; 3 mg iron; 0 mg cholesterol; 855 mg sodium.

Curried Chicken Salad

This main course salad is a delicious way to use leftover chicken. Or you can plan ahead and cook extra chicken to make this salad the next day.

SERVES 2 TO 4 AS A SNACK OR LIGHT MEAL, OR IN COMBINATION
WITH A SOUP, IT'S QUITE A FILLING MEAL

Lemon Curry Dressing

3 tablespoons extra virgin olive oil
3 tablespoons fresh lemon juice
3 tablespoons Virgin Coconut Oil Mayonnaise (page 208) or
 Simple Olive Oil Mayonnaise (page 168)*
2 teaspoons healthy low-carb sweetener (If using stevia or
 Lo Han Guo, less is needed.)
1 to 2 teaspoons curry powder
2 tablespoons chopped fresh basil or 1 to 2 teaspoons dried
½ teaspoon sea salt or Celtic salt (optional)

Chicken Salad

2 cups cooked chicken, skin removed, cut into bite-size pieces
3 cups romaine, green leaf, or Bibb lettuce, washed, dried, and
 torn into bite-size pieces
2 cups baby field greens (mesclun)
1 cup chopped cilantro
½ cup chopped red onion
¼ cup chopped green onions

In a small bowl, whisk together the dressing ingredients. Add the chicken to the dressing and toss to coat. Chill until ready to serve.

In a large salad bowl, combine the lettuces and greens, cilantro, and onions. Just before serving, add the chicken and dressing and toss.

*Be aware that many commercially made mayonnaise brands use soybean oil or other oils that are not part of this diet.

Nutritional breakdown per serving: 252 calories (42.7% from fat); 12 g fat; 29 g protein; 7 g carbohydrate; 1 g fiber; 69 mg cholesterol; 94 mg sodium.

SALAD DRESSINGS
TO MAKE ANY SALAD SPECIAL

Basic Vinaigrette

MAKES 1 CUP: ABOUT 16 SERVINGS

¼ cup red wine vinegar
Sea salt or Celtic salt, to taste
Black pepper, freshly ground
⅜ cup extra-virgin olive oil
⅜ cup virgin coconut oil (melted if solid)

In a small bowl, combine vinegar, salt, and pepper. Whisk until salt dissolves.

Combine olive oil and coconut oil until liquid is well blended.

Whisk in oil slowly, pouring in a slow, thin stream. Allow to stand 5 minutes. Whisk again, then taste and adjust seasonings, if needed.

Note: Basic dressing can be stored on the shelf or refrigerated, covered, up to one week. If refrigerated, warm to room temperature before using; whisk or shake just before using.

Nutritional breakdown per serving: 89 calories (99.0% from fat); 10 g fat; 0 g protein; trace carbohydrate; 0 g dietary fiber; 0 mg cholesterol; trace sodium.

Caper and Egg Vinaigrette

MAKES 1 CUP: ABOUT 16 SERVINGS

¼ cup red wine vinegar
Sea salt or Celtic salt, to taste
Black pepper, freshly ground
1 tablespoon capers, drained
2 tablespoons fresh parsley, chopped
⅜ cup extra-virgin olive oil
⅜ cup virgin coconut oil, melted if solid
1 egg, hard-boiled, finely chopped

In a small bowl, combine vinegar, salt, and pepper. Whisk until salt dissolves. Add capers and parsley.

Combine olive oil and coconut oil and stir until liquid.

Whisk in oil slowly in a slow, thin stream. Allow to stand 5 minutes. Whisk again, then taste and adjust seasonings, if needed. Stir in chopped egg.

Note: Basic dressing can be stored on shelf or refrigerated, covered, up to one week. Warm to room temperature and whisk before using.

Nutritional breakdown per serving: 94 calories (97.2% from fat); 11 g fat; trace protein; trace carbohydrate; trace dietary fiber; 13 mg cholesterol; 9 mg sodium.

Garlic Vinaigrette

MAKES 1 CUP: ABOUT 16 SERVINGS

⅜ cup extra-virgin olive oil
⅜ cup virgin coconut oil, melted if solid
½ tablespoon minced garlic
¼ cup red wine vinegar
Sea salt or Celtic salt
Black pepper, freshly ground

Combine olive oil and coconut oil and stir until liquid and well combined.

Cover minced garlic with ¾ cup combined oil and let stand 30 minutes.

In a small bowl, combine vinegar, salt, and pepper. Whisk until salt dissolves.

Whisk in oil slowly in a slow, thin stream. Allow to stand 5 minutes. Whisk again, then taste and adjust seasonings, if needed.

Note: Use dressing within a day or two. Can be stored on shelf or in refrigerator. If refrigerated, warm to room temperature; whisk before using.

Nutritional breakdown per serving: 90 calories (98.6% from fat); 10 g fat; trace protein; trace carbohydrate; trace dietary fiber; 0 mg cholesterol; trace sodium.

Lemon-Chive Vinaigrette

Makes 1 cup: about 16 servings

¼ cup fresh lemon juice
½ teaspoon lemon zest
Sea salt or Celtic salt
Black pepper, freshly ground
⅜ cup virgin coconut oil, melted if solid
⅜ cup extra-virgin olive oil
2 tablespoons minced fresh chives

In a small bowl, combine lemon juice, zest, salt, and pepper. Whisk until salt dissolves.

Combine coconut oil and olive oil and stir until liquid.

Whisk in oil slowly in a thin, steady stream, and allow to stand 5 minutes. Whisk again, then taste and adjust seasonings, if needed. Stir in minced chives.

Note: Basic dressing can be stored on shelf or refrigerated, covered, up to one week. Warm to room temperature and whisk before using.

Nutritional breakdown per serving: 90 calories (98.3% from fat); 10 g fat; trace protein; trace carbohydrate; trace dietary fiber; 0 mg cholesterol; trace sodium.

Mustard Vinaigrette

MAKES 1 CUP: ABOUT 16 SERVINGS

¼ cup red wine vinegar
2 teaspoons Dijon mustard
Sea salt or Celtic salt
Black pepper, freshly ground
⅜ cup virgin coconut oil, melted if solid
⅜ cup extra-virgin olive oil

In a small bowl, combine vinegar, Dijon mustard, salt, and pepper. Whisk until salt dissolves.

Combine coconut and olive oils and stir until liquid.

Whisk in oil slowly in a slow, thin stream, and allow to stand 5 minutes. Whisk again, then taste and adjust seasonings, if needed.

Note: Basic dressing can be stored on shelf or refrigerated, covered, up to one week. Warm to room temperature and whisk before using.

Nutritional breakdown per serving: 90 calories (98.8% from fat); 10 g fat; trace protein; trace carbohydrate; trace dietary fiber; 0 mg cholesterol; 8 mg sodium.

Tarragon Vinaigrette

MAKES 1 CUP: ABOUT 16 SERVINGS

¼ cup white wine vinegar
Sea salt or Celtic salt
Black pepper, freshly ground
⅜ cup extra-virgin olive oil
⅜ cup virgin coconut oil, melted if solid
1 tablespoon minced fresh tarragon or 1 to 2 teaspoons dried

In a small bowl, combine vinegar, salt, and pepper. Whisk until salt dissolves.

Combine olive and coconut oils and stir until liquid.

Whisk in oil slowly. Allow to stand 5 minutes. Whisk again, then taste and adjust seasonings, if needed. Stir in minced tarragon.

Note: Basic dressing can be stored on shelf or refrigerated, covered, up to one week. Whisk before using and allow to warm to room temperature.

Nutritional breakdown per serving: 89 calories (99.0% from fat); 10 g fat; 0 g protein; trace carbohydrate; 0 g dietary fiber; 0 mg cholesterol; trace sodium.

Tomato-Herb Vinaigrette

MAKES 1¼ CUPS: ABOUT 20 SERVINGS

2 tablespoons unsulfured apple cider vinegar
1 tablespoon fresh lemon juice
1 teaspoon Dijon mustard
2 tablespoons minced, fresh flat-leaf parsley
⅜ cup extra-virgin olive oil
⅜ cup virgin coconut oil, melted if solid
½ cup diced tomato
2 teaspoons minced fresh chives
Sea salt or Celtic salt
Black pepper, freshly ground

In a small bowl, whisk together vinegar, lemon juice, mustard, and parsley.

Combine olive and coconut oils and stir until liquid.

Add oil in a slow, steady stream, whisking constantly: mixture should be thick and creamy.

Stir in tomatoes and chives, and season with salt and pepper to taste. Use within a day or two.

Nutritional breakdown per serving: 73 calories (97.5% from fat); 8 g fat; trace protein; trace carbohydrate; trace dietary fiber; 0 mg cholesterol; 4 mg sodium.

SOUPS AND STEWS

Basic Gazpacho

This is a low-carb version of the classic gazpacho, without the bread-crumbs.

SERVES 8

3 pounds ripe tomatoes, peeled, seeded, and chopped
½ pound cucumbers, peeled, seeded, and chopped
1 cup chopped celery
½ cup chopped red bell pepper
½ cup red onion, chopped
1 teaspoon chopped garlic
1 tablespoon chopped jalapeño pepper
3 tablespoons red wine vinegar
¼ cup virgin coconut oil
12 ounces tomato juice
Salt, to taste
Freshly ground black pepper, to taste
Dash ground coriander
3 tablespoons chopped cilantro
1 lime, cut into slices

Gazpacho Relish

2 tablespoons small-diced red pepper
2 tablespoons small-diced cucumber
2 tablespoons small-diced red onion
2 tablespoons small-diced red tomatoes
1 teaspoon minced garlic
1 tablespoon lime juice
1 tablespoon extra-virgin olive oil
Salt, to taste
Freshly ground black pepper, to taste

Combine all ingredients in a blender or food processor except lime and puree until smooth.

Transfer to a large bowl and refrigerate for 4 hours.

In a small bowl, prepare the Gazpacho Relish by combining all ingredients. Ladle out soup into pretty bowls, top with a large tablespoon of relish and a slice of lime.

Nutritional breakdown per serving: 133 calories (55.8% from fat); 9 g fat; 2 g protein; 14 g carbohydrate; 3 g dietary fiber; 0 mg cholesterol; 183 mg sodium.

Thai Chicken Soup with Coconut and Galanga

This is as good as an authentic Thai restaurant coconut chicken soup.

MAKES 4 CUPS: 4 SERVINGS

1 tablespoon virgin coconut oil
1 medium shallot, sliced thin
1 garlic clove, minced
1½ tablespoons lemongrass, minced fine
2 chilies, sliced paper thin
1 teaspoon red curry paste
24 ounces chicken stock, preferably fresh
10 ounces coconut milk (if using canned, add all 13½ ounces of coconut milk and cut back a bit on the chicken stock)
1 (2-inch) piece galanga root,* sliced thin and bruised with the back of a knife
3 tablespoons Thai fish sauce
2 Roma tomatoes, seeded and diced
1 cup mushrooms, sliced into pie-shaped wedges
8 ounces skinless, boneless chicken breast, cut into ½-inch dice
4 Kaffir lime leaves, bruised
1 tablespoon lime juice, or to taste
2 tablespoons cilantro, shredded

Heat the oil in a heavy-bottomed, non-reactive pot. Add shallot, garlic, lemongrass, chilies, and red curry paste. Stir constantly for 30 seconds or until fragrant, but not colored.

Add chicken stock, coconut milk, galanga root (or ginger root), and fish sauce. Bring the pot to a boil, then reduce heat and simmer 3 minutes.

Add tomatoes, mushrooms, chicken, and Kaffir lime leaves. Bring the pot back to a simmer and simmer very gently for 5 minutes.

Add lime juice, and remove the pot from heat. Remove galanga and Kaffir lime leaves; garnish with cilantro, as desired, and serve.

*Galanga is a member of the ginger root family and the primary ginger used in Thai cooking; it's available in Asian markets. If unavailable, substitute ginger root.

Nutritional breakdown per serving: 346 calories (61.3% from fat); 24 g fat; 17 g protein; 16 g carbohydrate; 3 g dietary fiber; 35 mg cholesterol; 95 mg sodium.

Turkey Stew

Make this stew for dinner and serve a bowl up for lunch the next day.

MAKES 12 CUPS: 6 SERVINGS

1½ pounds turkey thighs, skin removed
5 cups water to cover (5 to 6 cups)
2 bay leaves
5 peppercorns
3 sprigs parsley
1 stalk celery, cut into 1-inch chunks
1 cup jicama, cut into ½-inch cubes
1 large onion, cut in half and quartered
1 large carrot, peeled and cut into ½-inch slices
1 (14-ounce) can tomatoes, drained
1 (10-ounce) package frozen okra

1½ teaspoons sea salt or Celtic salt
1 teaspoon minced garlic
½ teaspoon coarsely ground pepper
½ teaspoon dried oregano
⅛ teaspoon mace
1 cup wild rice, cooked according to package directions

In 5-quart saucepan over high heat, bring to boil turkey thighs, water, bay leaves, peppercorns, parsley, and celery. Cover, reduce heat, and simmer for 45 minutes.

Remove and discard bay leaves and parsley. Remove thighs and allow to cool enough to handle. Remove meat from the bone and cut into large chunks. Discard bones.

Return turkey to pan along with jicama, onion, carrot, tomatoes, okra, salt, garlic, pepper, oregano, and mace. Bring to a boil; reduce heat and simmer 30 minutes or until vegetables are tender.

Stir in cooked wild rice and serve in soup bowls.

Nutritional breakdown per serving: 379 calories (27.9% from fat); 12 g fat; 37 g protein; 31 g carbohydrate; 5 g dietary fiber; 96 mg cholesterol; 908 mg sodium.

VEGETABLE DISHES

Tasty Greens Sauté

The following recipe can be applied to most green leafy vegetables: Swiss chard, kale, collard greens, beet tops, spinach, and so forth. A mixture of several of them, or just one, especially spinach, could readily be used in this way. A wok-type pan may be found most useful for stir-frying these vegetables. Wash the greens and dry them.

SERVES 4

3 tablespoons virgin coconut oil
½ teaspoon cumin seeds
1 large yellow onion, sliced or chopped
1 cup mushrooms, sliced

½ teaspoon clove powder
1 teaspoon turmeric powder
1 teaspoon coriander powder
1 to 2 garlic cloves, crushed
8 to 10 cups of greens (Swiss chard, kale, collard greens, beet tops,
    spinach, torn into bits, if large)
1 cup feta cheese, crumbled into small lumps
¼ cup fresh lime juice

Gently heat oil and cumin seeds.

Add the onion and about 5 minutes later the mushrooms, stirring frequently.

Add the spices and garlic, stirring all the while.

Add the greens and mix everything together well. Keep stirring until the greens are wilted (limp).

Add the feta cheese and let it melt into the greens and drizzle some fresh lime juice over it all. The whole process will take only 10 to 15 minutes.

Serving suggestions: This dish makes an excellent accompaniment for an omelet, which would make this a meal that can be produced in just a few minutes, and could be a great brunch item. It also goes well with any other kind of protein.

Nutritional breakdown per serving: 363 calories (55% from fat); 24 g fat; 14 g protein; 30 g carbohydrate; 8 g fiber; 443 mg calcium; 5 mg iron; 33 mg cholesterol; 1,272 mg sodium.

Artichokes with Hollandaise Sauce

These artichokes are delicious served with Classic Blender Hollandaise Sauce (page 160) or with Aioli (page 208) or other flavored mayonnaise.

SERVES 4

4 large artichokes
1 lemon, quartered

Trim artichokes for steaming or boiling by trimming top and stems and trimming thorns from leaves.

Steam artichokes until tender and leaves pull freely or boil in salted water for 35 to 45 minutes.

Serve each artichoke with a lemon quarter and your favorite sauce.

Nutritional breakdown per serving (figured with hollandaise sauce): 313 calories (72.9% from fat); 27 g fat; 7 g protein; 16 g carbohydrate; 7 g dietary fiber; 222 mg cholesterol; 129 mg sodium.

Classic Blender Hollandaise Sauce

This hollandaise sauce is so easy to make and is delicious.

MAKES 6 OUNCES: ABOUT 12 SERVINGS

3 large egg yolks, whole
2 tablespoons fresh lemon juice
Dash cayenne pepper
4 ounces unsalted butter, melted and bubbling hot

In a blender, combine egg yolks, lemon juice, and cayenne pepper and blend on high speed for 3 seconds.

Remove lid and with motor running, slowly pour hot butter in a steady stream over eggs. When butter is all poured in, blend an additional 5 seconds.

Taste and adjust seasonings to taste.

Serve immediately or keep sauce warm by placing blender in a bowl of warm water.

Nutritional breakdown per serving: 83 calories (94.8% from fat); 9 g fat; 1 g protein; trace carbohydrate; trace dietary fiber; 74 mg cholesterol; 3 mg sodium.

DINNER RECIPES

Chicken with Citrus-Garlic-Ginger Sauce

This dish offers a delicious burst of citrus flavor.

SERVES 4

3½-pound chicken, disjointed and breasts de-boned or 1 chicken
    precut
Sea salt or Celtic salt, to taste
Black pepper, freshly ground, to taste
3 to 4 tablespoons virgin coconut oil
1 tablespoon garlic, minced
1 tablespoon fresh ginger, peeled and minced
1 tablespoon lemon zest
1 tablespoon lime zest
1 cup chicken stock, preferably fresh

Disjoint chicken thighs and legs and de-bone breasts, reserving carcass and wings for chicken stock, if using a whole chicken, or use precut chicken; reserve wings and neck for a nice chicken broth for other recipes.

Season chicken pieces with salt and pepper on both sides to taste.

Heat 2 tablespoons coconut oil in sauté pan over medium-high heat until shimmering.

Brown chicken pieces on all sides until golden brown and set aside (chicken will not be done).

Add garlic, ginger, and citrus zests to pan, tossing until softened and fragrant.

Deglaze pan with chicken stock, scraping up browned bits in pan. Return chicken to pan, cover, and simmer over low heat until chicken breasts reach 165 degrees F (75 degrees C) and thighs and legs reach 175 degrees F (80 degrees C). Remove chicken to serving platter as pieces reach target temperature.

After all the chicken is cooked, finish the sauce by swirling in 1 to 2 tablespoons virgin coconut oil. Pour sauce over chicken and reserve some to drizzle over spinach and/or wild rice.

Serve over steamed spinach or wild rice.*

*Wild rice is a grass, not a grain, and it is lower in carbs than rice. It is permitted in Phase I in small amounts; about a ¼-cup serving, which yields about 9 grams of carbs.

Nutritional breakdown per serving: 602 calories (69.8% from fat); 46 g fat; 43 g protein; 1 g carbohydrate; trace dietary fiber; 226 mg cholesterol; 174 mg sodium.

Chili

This is an American favorite, but keep in mind that a bowl of chili will provide about one serving of legumes (beans) for the week.

MAKES 6 SERVINGS

1 large yellow onion, chopped
1 green pepper, chopped
2 tablespoons virgin coconut oil
1 pound ground beef or turkey
2 (1 pound) cans (4 cups) tomatoes
1 to 2 teaspoons chili powder
1½ teaspoons sea salt or Celtic salt
3 large cloves garlic, finely chopped
1 bay leaf
Dash of paprika
Dash of cayenne pepper
1 No. 2 can (2½ cups) red chili beans
¼ cup water, as desired

In a large soup kettle or Dutch oven, sauté onion and green pepper in coconut oil until tender, about 5 minutes on medium heat.

Add ground beef or turkey and cook until done. Add tomatoes and seasonings. Turn heat to low and simmer for 2 hours.

Add beans and heat thoroughly. Add water, as necessary.

Nutritional breakdown per serving: 485 calories (39% from fat); 21 g fat; 29 g protein; 47 g carbohydrate; 18 g dietary fiber; 64 mg cholesterol; 617 mg sodium.

Healthy Hamburgers

Hamburgers without buns are the low-carb craze these days. Here's a variation you may not have thought about. Using a large lettuce leaf for each hamburger patty, spread a lettuce leaf out on each plate. Top the lettuce with sliced sweet onion (Vidalia onion is particularly sweet, but purple onion is nice, too), a slice of tomato, and some mustard of your choice. If necessary, use a second leaf of lettuce to wrap the hamburger, held in place with a toothpick or two, so that you can eat it as finger food. (Be careful not to bite into the toothpick when you start eating.) If not having it as finger food, omit the toothpicks, place it on a plate, and eat it with a fork and knife.

SERVES 4

1 pound ground beef or buffalo
1 teaspoon ground coriander
1 teaspoon ground cumin
1 teaspoon dried marjoram or 1 tablespoon fresh, minced
½ teaspoon paprika
½ teaspoon turmeric
½ teaspoon sea salt or Celtic salt
¼ teaspoon black pepper, freshly ground
1 teaspoon finely minced fresh garlic
2 free-range eggs
3 tablespoons virgin coconut oil
½ head lettuce (Boston, romaine, Bibb, etc.)
1 sweet Vidalia onion or red onion
1 tomato
Mustard, to taste

Place the meat in a bowl; add the spices and garlic (*do not* use garlic powder, it doesn't give the right flavor) and eggs.

Mix everything together well and form patties the size you wish.

Place patties in a pan in which the coconut oil has been melting (there should be a slight sizzle as the patties drop in).

Fry them slowly on both sides to make sure the meat is cooked completely through. Test one piece by breaking it open. There should be nothing pink inside. Lift the patties out and put them on paper towels to absorb any excess fat.

Top with lettuce, onion, tomato, and mustard.

Variation: Substitute ground lamb or turkey for an equally pleasing result.

Nutritional breakdown per serving: 396 calories (61% from fat); 27 g fat; 29 g protein; 10 g carbohydrate; 3 g fiber; 84 mg calcium; 5 mg iron; 192 mg cholesterol; 118 mg sodium.

Fish in Fennel Sauce

This recipe calls for a pound or two of fish. This can be a whole small fish (like rainbow trout) or it could be a number of fish steaks, or filets, fresh or frozen or whatever you have on hand. Its flavor will be immensely improved by marinating the fish for a day, covered in the refrigerator. Serve the fish and sauce over a bed of steamed green beans or wild rice. A salad of crisp greens, either Boston or romaine lettuce, with a lemony vinaigrette makes a nice complement.

SERVES 2

Marinade

1 tablespoon grated ginger
1 tablespoon grated lemon rind
Juice of 1 or 2 limes (depending on juiciness)
½ teaspoon turmeric powder

½ teaspoon sea salt or Celtic salt
1 pound of fish: filets, steaks, or whole fish*

Combine the marinade ingredients and rub them into the fish.

Put the fish into a covered dish (preferably glass or porcelain, not plastic) and keep it in the fridge overnight or for 24 hours.

Additional Ingredients for Sautéing

1 large yellow onion, sliced
1 medium fennel bulb, sliced
3 to 4 tablespoons virgin coconut oil
Sea salt or Celtic salt, to taste
Freshly ground black pepper, to taste
1 tablespoon capers

Coarsely slice the onion and the fennel bulb (stalks and greens included).

Remove fish from the marinade. You will notice that some yellow liquid will have formed. Keep it and add it later as the fish is cooking. Pat the fish dry.

Using enough coconut oil to cover the bottom of a pan, gently fry the fish on one side for just a few minutes and then turn it over. Put aside.

Add the onions and fennel to the pan and sauté for a few minutes and add the marinade liquid. Place the fish on top of the vegetables, cover the pan and cook for a short while. The time depends on the fish size. For example, a whole fish should cook about 15 minutes. The fish should not look glassy, but should be opaque inside.

Remove from heat and let stand, covered, for another 10 minutes. Check to see if there is sufficient seasoning, adding a pinch of salt and pepper as needed.

Sprinkle the capers over the fish last.

*If using frozen fish, there is no need to defrost it first. It can do so while marinating.

Nutritional breakdown per serving: 390 calories (46% from fat); 21 g fat; 27 g protein; 30 g carbohydrate; 10 g fiber; 158 mg calcium; 4 mg iron; 50 mg cholesterol; 329 mg sodium.

Golden Chicken

Chicken cooked in this manner is equally tasty cold, served with a salad, and, particularly where drumsticks are used, as a "finger food" for snacks.

SERVES 2 TO 4

4 chicken legs (add extra if preparing for lunch the next day or snacks)
1 teaspoon turmeric
1 teaspoon coriander
½ teaspoon cinnamon
½ teaspoon sea salt or Celtic salt
¼ to ½ cup fresh lemon juice
1 tablespoon coconut cream concentrate or virgin coconut oil

Preheat oven to medium heat, approximately 350 degrees F.

Wash the chicken* and pat it dry with a paper towel. Cut off any visible fat.

In a small bowl prepare the mixture of spices: turmeric, coriander, cinnamon, and salt. Using a sieve, dust the chicken pieces on both sides.

Use a rack (a cake rack works well) that will fit over a large pan and place the chicken pieces on it.

Bake for at least an hour. The meat should be cooked through and golden brown. Using this method will ensure that you get rid of most of the unwanted fat the chicken may have. It will simply drip into the tray below. The regular, supermarket-type chickens have a lot of fat, whereas organic free-range chickens tend to be more lean.

Toward the latter part of the baking, drizzle some lemon juice over the chicken. Do this once or twice. It will add a lovely flavor to the meat itself and the juice that is dripping away.

When cooked to satisfaction, lift the chicken off the rack and pour the fat and all juices into a shallow dish. Put the dish in the fridge or freezer where the fat will congeal; it can then be lifted off, leaving just the meat juice, which will form a gelatinous glob that can be warmed up again and drizzled over the meat. When this mixture is warmed, add the coconut cream or oil.

On use of spices: Turmeric will put a "golden glow" on almost any dish, but particularly on poultry. It is a spice almost devoid of any flavor of its own but has a way of improving the flavor of any dish.

*If using free-range chicken there is an enormous difference in the fat content. This type of bird tends to be lean and may, in fact, have hardly any fat on it at all. In this case rub the chicken with coconut cream or the coconut oil.

Nutritional breakdown per serving: 108 calories (48% from fat); 6 g fat; 12 g protein; 2 g sat fat; 2 g mono fat; 2 g carbohydrate; 1 g fiber; 12 mg calcium; 1 mg iron; 50 mg cholesterol; 52 mg sodium.

Chicken in Coconut Milk with Lime Leaves

Serve over a bed of steamed asparagus or steamed spinach, drained, or wild rice with a crisp green salad. A useful hint: Don't keep coconut milk in the fridge many days; it is perishable. Freeze it in ice cube trays and then store in a container (labeled accordingly) in the freezer.

SERVES 4

1 (13.5-ounce) can coconut milk (divide into two parts)
1 tablespoon Coconut Cream Concentrate (optional) (see Resources)
1 large yellow onion, diced
¼ teaspoon turmeric powder
¼ teaspoon coriander powder
1 teaspoon sea salt or Celtic salt
1 teaspoon fresh ginger root, finely diced
1 teaspoon fresh garlic, finely diced
1 stalk fresh lemongrass or lemon balm*
3 or 4 fresh lime leaves*
3 skinless chicken breasts, cut in chunks
1 fennel bulb, finely sliced

Use one-half of the coconut milk or enough to cover the bottom of the pan, add the coconut cream, as desired, and onion and cook for 3 minutes.

Add the spices, including the lemongrass and lime leaves, and cook for another minute or two.

Now add the chicken and the remainder of the coconut milk, cover well, and cook for about 20 minutes. Start out on high heat, then lower to medium-low heat to a "comfortable bubble."

Add the sliced fennel bulb, cover again, and cook for another 5 minutes. The fennel should still be a little al dente, or chewy, not totally soft.

*Lemongrass and lime leaves can be found in Asian specialty stores. If unable to find either, cut some strips of a fresh lime peel and finely chop (lime zest). Most stores have dried lemongrass, but it won't be as good as the fresh lemongrass. What you really want to get is the combination of the delicate sourness of lime leaves and lemongrass and the mellowness of coconut milk. Fresh lemon balm, an herb that's often locally grown, has almost the same flavor as lemongrass and can be substituted. Cut lemongrass in half to fit the pot, and remove it before serving.

Nutritional breakdown per serving: 395 calories (59% from fat); 27 g fat; 19 g protein; 23 g carbohydrate; 6 g fiber; 102 mg calcium; 6 mg iron; 33 mg cholesterol; 122 mg sodium.

Stuffed Rainbow Trout Filets

Trout is a rich source of omega-3 fatty acids, one of those good fats we all need to eat more often. With the low-carb stuffing, it's a special treat.

SERVES 4

Stuffing

1 pound fresh spinach (about 1½ packets) or 1 (10-ounce) package frozen spinach

2 cups mushrooms, sliced
½ cup finely sliced yellow onions
4 tablespoons virgin coconut oil
1 teaspoon allspice
1 teaspoon nutmeg
½ teaspoon sea salt or Celtic salt

Fish

4 large rainbow trout filets
Dash sea salt or Celtic salt, or to taste
½ teaspoon black pepper, freshly ground
½ cup fresh lime juice
4 (8-inch) lengths of cotton string (cut to measure)
2 cups pearl onions
2 cups water plus 2 tablespoons fresh lemon juice; divided
   (dry white wine can be substituted in Phase III)
1 tablespoon capers

Preheat oven to 350 degrees F.

Wash the spinach and pat it dry (spread it on a fresh towel and roll it up, patting it a few times. This is a quick way of getting it or other greens ready for sautéing). Discard the stems if they are large. If the spinach leaves are very large, chop them up a bit.

Wipe the mushrooms with a moist cloth and slice. Slice the onions thinly.

In a large pan, melt the coconut oil and quickly sauté the onions and mushrooms. Sprinkle with the ground allspice, nutmeg, and salt.

Add the spinach and stir-fry it just long enough to make it wilt. Set it aside.

Sprinkle the filets with a little salt, pepper, and lime juice.

Lay one filet flat on a board and put a generous helping of the spinach mixture on it, about 1 to 2 inches high. Place the second filet on top.

Use the string to tie the filets together to ensure that the stuffing stays inside while the fish is cooking.

Slide the string under the bottom filet at each end. Make sure the string is far enough from each end that you can secure it properly. Loop it around, pull it up, and tie a knot. This method is much better than trying to use toothpicks to secure the pieces.

Prepare a baking dish (heat-proof glass or Corningware—ready-to-serve is best) by generously brushing or rubbing it with coconut oil.

Place the filets in the dish surrounded by the pearl onions and a cup of lemon water (dry white wine can be used when you progress to Phase III).

Bake for about 30 to 40 minutes, basting it from time to time to prevent the top layer from drying out.

Finally, pour the baking liquid into a saucepan, add the other cup of lemon water (or dry white wine) and cook it over high heat to reduce it quickly to a thick sauce. Add the capers. Remove the string from the filets, pour the sauce over them, and serve.

Nutritional breakdown per serving: 328 calories (46% from fat); 16 g fat; 23 g protein; 18 g carbohydrate; 5 g fiber; 219 mg calcium; 3 mg iron; 48 mg cholesterol; 572 mg sodium.

Lamb and Eggplant Casserole

In Phase III, serve with a dollop of plain yogurt, especially when adding some hot spices or pepper sauce; the yogurt will be cooling. For a spicy dish, add some cayenne pepper along with the other ground spices. The bits of red or yellow pepper will add a dash of bright color.

SERVES 4 OR MORE

1 teaspoon cumin seeds
3 tablespoons virgin coconut oil
2 cups chopped onions
1 teaspoon turmeric
1 teaspoon ground coriander
½ teaspoon ground allspice

½ teaspoon ground cloves
1 tablespoon crushed fresh garlic
1½ pounds ground lamb
2 to 3 medium-sized eggplants, cubed
1 red and 1 yellow pepper, coarsely chopped
1 to 2 teaspoons sea salt or Celtic salt

In a pot or wok pan, toast (dry cook) the cumin seeds to elicit a nice aroma from them.

Add the coconut oil and the onions. Keep stirring until the onions are translucent.

Add the ground spices: turmeric, coriander, allspice, and cloves.

Add the crushed garlic and keep stirring.

Add the ground lamb, stir well, and cook until the meat no longer looks pink, for about 5 minutes.

Add the cubed eggplants and the coarsely chopped peppers. Cover the pot or pan and braise for about 15 to 20 minutes.

Sprinkle salt to taste and let it stand for a few minutes before serving.

Regarding braising: An easy alternative to this procedure is to combine all the ingredients in a casserole dish, put the dish in the oven and bake it for about 45 to 60 minutes at moderate heat (325 to 350 degrees F).

Nutritional breakdown per serving: 703 calories (53% from fat); 42 g fat; 48 g protein; 36 g carbohydrate; 12 g fiber; 105 mg calcium; 6 mg iron; 165 mg cholesterol; 188 mg sodium.

Salmon Steaks with Vegetables

For those of you who dislike washing dishes, try cooking food in one pot, pan, or wok. Not only does this cut down on the number of utensils used, but by combining protein and plant foods in one vessel, the flavor of all the foods is enhanced. Food actually tastes much better cooked this way. This dish goes well with a crispy green salad.

SERVES 4

**1 medium yellow onion, finely sliced
1 medium yellow onion, coarsely sliced
2 cups yellow summer squash, sliced
1 large red pepper, coarsely sliced
4 tablespoons virgin coconut oil
½ teaspoon turmeric
½ teaspoon coriander
½ teaspoon sea salt or Celtic Salt
4 salmon steaks
1 tablespoon fresh oregano or marjoram, chopped, or ½ tablespoon dried
1 tablespoon fresh lime or lemon juice**

Chop one onion finely, and the other very coarsely, into about 1-inch squares. Slice the squash and peppers very coarsely.

Heat the oil in a pan; use a wok, Dutch oven, or skillet with a good strong base. There should be little bubbles forming on the bottom of the pan before adding the vegetables.

Add the onions and cook for about 10 minutes or until tender; then add the squash and the peppers.

Next add the turmeric, coriander, and salt.

Stir-fry for about 10 minutes, then push the vegetables aside and put the salmon steaks in the center of the pan.

Sear the underside for about 3 minutes and turn them over. Arrange the vegetables on top of the salmon, add the herbs and a sprinkling of lime or lemon, and cover the pan or Dutch oven with a well-fitting lid.

Reduce the heat and cook for about 5 minutes, or until fish is opaque in center.

Nutritional breakdown per serving: 865 calories (49% from fat); 46 g fat; 82 g protein; 9 g sat fat; 17 g mono fat; 27 g carbohydrate; 4 g fiber; 99 mg cholesterol; 236 mg sodium.

Super-Speedy Supper

There are times when something healthy is needed really fast. This is one of those dishes. And nothing is nicer to go with this supper than a juicy, crunchy salad such as fresh tomatoes, cucumbers, radishes, green onions, and a favorite greens with a dressing of lemon juice and a dash of olive oil or a vinaigrettes (pages 172–176).

Serves 4

2 tablespoons virgin coconut oil
1 teaspoon cumin seeds
1 pound ground beef, buffalo, lamb, turkey, or chicken
½ medium cabbage, shredded
1 medium yellow onion, chopped
1 teaspoon paprika
1 teaspoon nutmeg
1 tablespoon crushed garlic
2 tablespoon green olives, sliced
1 tablespoon finely chopped fresh parsley

Heat the oil in a pan and add the cumin seeds and ground meat. Stir-fry for about 5 minutes, or until meat has no pink.

Add the shredded cabbage, onion, paprika, nutmeg, crushed garlic, and olives. Mix well and stir-fry for another 5 minutes.

Garnish with parsley.

Nutritional breakdown per serving: 279 calories (57% from fat); 18 g fat; 23 g protein; 7 g carbohydrate; 2 g fiber; 69 mg cholesterol; 107 mg sodium.

Lemon Tarragon Fish

Serve over a bed of wild rice with steamed asparagus and globe arti-chokes.

SERVES 2

½ teaspoon turmeric powder
½ teaspoon paprika
½ teaspoon curry powder
½ teaspoon cinnamon
½ teaspoon sea salt or Celtic salt
2 filets cod or Boston bluefish
3 to 4 tablespoons virgin coconut oil
2 large yellow onions, sliced
2 large tomatoes, sliced
Dash of sea salt or Celtic salt
1 teaspoon dried tarragon or 2 teaspoons fresh, chopped
3 tablespoons fresh lemon juice

Preheat oven to 350 degrees F.

Mix the spices and rub them on the filets on both sides.

Prepare a baking dish by rubbing it generously with coconut oil.

Spread the sliced onions on the bottom of the dish, followed by the sliced tomatoes, a sprinkling of salt, and dried or fresh tarragon, and finally the fish.

Drizzle the lemon juice over top.

Bake the fish for about 35 minutes or until opaque in the center, basting it with the pan juices from time to time.

Nutritional breakdown per serving: 456 calories (30% from fat); 13 g fat; 45 g protein; 23 g carbohydrate; 5 g fiber; 99 mg cholesterol; 167 mg sodium.

Stuffed Beef Rolls

Apart from serving this dish warm and fresh, these roll-ups are quite delicious served cold. Slice them up and hand them out as an appetizer or as a quick light meal with a salad; one containing sauerkraut is especially good.

SERVES 4 TO 6

4 flank steaks
1 tablespoon Dijon mustard
4 slices pastrami
4 green onions, halved
1 large carrot, quartered lengthwise
1 large dill pickle, quartered lengthwise
2 tablespoons fresh marjoram, chopped, or 1 tablespoon dried
4 (8-inch) lengths of cotton string (cut as required)
3 tablespoons virgin coconut oil
2 cups chopped yellow onions
½ teaspoon sea salt or Celtic salt
½ teaspoon black pepper, freshly ground
1 (approximately 12-ounce) can stewed tomatoes
1 to 2 cups whole small mushrooms

Pound the flank steaks with a mallet or meat tenderizer.

Lay them flat on a cutting board and thinly spread some Dijon mustard on each of the steaks. Next place a slice of pastrami on each.

Cut up the green onions to fit the width of the steak. Place a green onion on one end, followed by a strip of carrot and dill pickle (simply cut it into 4 lengths to fit the width of the flank steak).

Sprinkle with the dried or fresh marjoram and then roll up each steak, securing it with the cotton string.

Melt the coconut oil and lightly brown the meat on all sides.

Add the chopped onions and cook until they turn a nice golden color, add salt and pepper, the can of stewed tomatoes, and the mushrooms. If small mushrooms are not available, then use large ones and cut them in quarters.

Cover and cook on moderate to low heat for about an hour. Check the pan during that time to ensure that there is enough liquid in it. If necessary, add a little water. Test the meat to make sure it is cooked through and tender enough to be served. If thicker sauce is desired, remove the meat and quickly reduce the liquid by cooking it on very high heat, stirring constantly. This will only take a minute or two.

Nutritional breakdown per serving: 932 calories (44% from fat); 45 g fat; 98 g protein; 32 g carbohydrate; 7 g fiber; 241 mg cholesterol; 1,497 mg sodium.

Baked Lemon Chicken Thighs

This dish is nice served with a combination of steamed vegetables and crispy garden salad, or the Steamed Vegetable Salad (page 169).

Serves 4

1 teaspoon turmeric
1 teaspoon coriander
½ teaspoon sea salt or Celtic salt
½ teaspoon black pepper, freshly ground
8 chicken thighs
3 tablespoons virgin coconut oil
2 cups pearl onions
¼ cup fresh lemon juice

Mix turmeric, coriander, salt, and pepper.

Rub the chicken thighs with the spice mixture.

In a pan, heat the oil and add the chicken thighs. Fry gently until they are golden brown on both sides.

Add the pearl onions (if substitute is needed use regular yellow or cooking onions, but chop them coarsely). Cook for another 10 minutes.

Add the lemon juice, cover the pan, reduce heat to low (a "comfortable bubble"), and cook for another 15 minutes. At this point the chicken should be tender and dripping with a delicate, lemony flavor.

Nutritional breakdown per serving: 281 calories (60% from fat); 19 g fat; 20 g protein; 8 g carbohydrate; 2 g fiber; 69 mg cholesterol; 487 mg sodium.

Marinated Steak

These steaks are nice served with a crunchy salad made of romaine lettuce, finely sliced celery, radishes, and cherry tomatoes.

SERVES 2

2 steaks such as tenderloin or New York strip
⅔ cup apple cider vinegar
¼ cup tamari or soy sauce
2 tablespoons virgin coconut oil
2 red peppers, cored and cut in chunks
1 large yellow onion, cut in chunks
½ teaspoon black pepper, freshly ground

Place the steaks in a glass or porcelain (not plastic) dish and pour the apple cider vinegar and tamari (or soy) sauce over them. Let them marinate in the fridge for 8 hours.

Lift the steaks out of the marinade and pat them dry. Discard the marinade.

Heat the coconut oil in a pan and place the steaks in it. Fry for about 3 minutes on one side and turn them over.

Add the peppers and onion (separate the various layers), then add the black pepper.

Cover with a lid and cook for another 3 minutes. This will create some delicious pan juices, which can be spooned over steamed vegetables.

Note: There may be no need for additional salt since both the tamari and soy sauce tends to be quite salty.

Nutritional breakdown per serving: 811 calories (47% from fat); 43 g fat; 84 g protein; 24 g carbohydrate; 5 g fiber; 221 mg cholesterol; 2,208 mg sodium.

Turkey in Coconut Milk

Wild rice and a salad of finely sliced cucumbers, celery, and lettuce with a lemon dressing go nicely with this dish.

SERVES 4 TO 8 (DEPENDING ON SIZE OF TURKEY THIGHS)

4 turkey thighs
4 tablespoons virgin coconut oil
1 large onion, coarsely chopped
3 to 4 green chilies, seeded, chopped (optional)
1 teaspoon cumin seeds
6 cloves garlic, finely chopped
1 cup chicken or turkey stock, divided
¼ cup fresh lemon juice
1 cup coconut milk, divided
½ teaspoon crushed dried rosemary

Sauté the turkey thighs in 3 tablespoons of the oil until golden, turning it on all sides. Transfer to an ovenproof dish.

Add the remaining 1 tablespoon of oil to the pan, and sauté the onions, chilies (optional), and cumin seed until the onions are golden.

Add the chopped garlic and continue cooking, making sure that the garlic is not fried, roasted, or burned.

Cover the turkey with the onion mixture.

Deglaze the pan with ½ cup of chicken or turkey stock and pour into the casserole dish.

Combine the remaining ½ cup of stock, lemon juice, ½ cup coconut milk, and the rosemary and add to the casserole. Cover and bake at 325 to 350 degrees F until the meat is very tender, about 1½ hours.

Remove the meat to a hot platter and keep warm.

Reduce the contents of the casserole by cooking it over high heat until the sauce is quite thick.

Add the remaining ½ cup of coconut milk and heat through. Pour the sauce over the meat.

Nutritional breakdown per serving: 477 calories (70% from fat); 39 g fat; 25 g protein; 11 g carbohydrate; 2 g fiber; 66 mg cholesterol; 327 mg sodium.

Baked Drumsticks with Spicy Eggplant

Anything cooked with eggplant will taste better the next day, as it readily absorbs spices and juices.

SERVES 4 TO 6

2 large eggplants, sliced lengthwise
3 tablespoons virgin coconut oil
1 teaspoon cumin seeds
½ teaspoon cumin powder
1 teaspoon turmeric
½ teaspoon coriander powder
1 teaspoon sea salt or Celtic salt
8 to 10 chicken drumsticks
½ cup fresh lemon juice

Preheat oven to about 350 degrees F.

Peel the eggplants if they are very large, otherwise just slice them lengthwise into about half-inch-thick slices.

Prepare a baking dish by rubbing or brushing it generously with the coconut oil; sprinkle with the cumin seeds.

Mix the spices together and sprinkle over the eggplant slices and the drumsticks.

Place the eggplant slices into the baking dish and cover them with drumsticks. Depending on the size of the baking dish and drumsticks, you may need to remove a drumstick or two.

Cover everything with the lemon juice and put it in the oven. Bake for an hour or until the drumsticks are properly cooked through the center and the eggplant has been reduced to a creamy, mushy consistency.

Nutritional breakdown per serving: 306 calories (38% from fat); 13 g fat; 33 g protein; 14 g carbohydrate; 5 g fiber; 107 mg cholesterol; 124 mg sodium.

Chicken Breasts in Chunky Tomato-Vegetable Sauce

This is an exceedingly easy and quick-to-make dish, using only one pan, and makes a lovely rich broth that includes vegetables. The chicken and vegetables will produce a delicious flavor, but it is imperative to keep the moisture in the pan, using a well-fitting lid or foil. Note the absence of water, which would only serve to dilute the rich flavor.

SERVES 4

½ teaspoon turmeric
½ teaspoon curry powder
½ teaspoon paprika
½ teaspoon cinnamon
4 chicken breasts, skinned
3 tablespoons virgin coconut oil
½ teaspoon sea salt or Celtic salt
1 red pepper, sliced
1 yellow onion, coarsely cut in chunks
3 plum tomatoes, chopped
1 cup fresh herbs or ½ cup dried herbs
¼ cup fresh lime or lemon juice

In a small bowl blend the spices and, using a small sieve, dust the chicken with this spice mixture.

Arrange chicken on a cutting board.

Heat coconut oil in a frying pan until it forms tiny bubbles. There should be a slight sizzle when placing the pieces of chicken into the pan. Allow them to turn a lovely golden color before turning them over.

Sprinkle some salt over the chicken breasts and then cover them with the red pepper, onion, tomatoes, and fresh or dried herbs such as thyme, marjoram, or tarragon or any other so desired. (If only dried herbs are available, choose some favorites.)

Cover the pan with a well-fitting lid and reduce the heat to a simmer for about 30 minutes, or until the chicken is completely done (opaque in the center).

When chicken is completely cooked, drizzle some fresh lime or lemon juice over the dish.

Nutritional breakdown per serving: 249 calories (54% from fat), 16 g fat, 18 g protein; 12 g carbohydrate; 4 g fiber; 43 mg cholesterol; 49 mg sodium.

Sautéed Chicken Breasts with Pico de Gallo

A nice south-of-the border flavor that tastes as if it took considerable time, but the good news is that it's very easy to prepare.

Serves 4

4 (6-ounce) skinless, boneless chicken breasts
Sea salt or Celtic salt, to taste
Black pepper, freshly ground
1 tablespoon virgin coconut oil
4 tablespoons Pico de Gallo (page 204)

Preheat oven to 350 degrees F.

Gently pound chicken breast pieces to thickness of ⅜ to ½ inch for consistent cooking.

Season chicken breasts with salt and pepper on both sides.

In a stainless steel skillet, over medium-high heat, melt coconut oil until shimmering.

Add chicken breasts and sauté until golden brown, about 4 to 6 minutes.

Turn over and brown the other side, about 4 to 6 minutes.

Bake for 6 to 10 minutes, until internal temperature is 165 degrees F (74 degrees C).

Place on plate and spoon Pico de Gallo on top.

Nutritional breakdown per serving: 221 calories (23.6% from fat); 6 g fat; 39 g protein; 1 g carbohydrate; trace dietary fiber; 99 mg cholesterol; 112 mg sodium.

Pico de Gallo

This will also make a nice salad dressing or dip for veggie sticks.

MAKES 2 CUPS: ABOUT 32 SERVINGS

1 pound tomatoes, diced
1 medium yellow onion, diced
6 tablespoons fresh cilantro (packed), chopped
2 tablespoons fresh lime juice
1 teaspoon fresh lime zest
2 large garlic cloves, minced
1 large jalapeño, seeded and minced

Toss all ingredients in a medium bowl until well blended. Refrigerate until ready for use.

Nutritional breakdown per serving: 5 calories (8.4% calories from fat); trace fat; trace protein; 1 g carbohydrate; trace dietary fiber; 0 mg cholesterol; 1 mg sodium.

Sautéed Chicken Breasts with Tomato Sauce

This dish is nice served over a bed of steamed spinach or wild rice.

SERVES 4

4 (6-ounce) skinless boneless chicken breasts
Sea salt or Celtic salt, to taste
Black pepper, freshly ground
1 tablespoon virgin coconut oil
4 to 8 tablespoons Tomato Sauce (page 206)

Preheat oven to 350 degrees F.

Gently pound chicken breast pieces to same thickness, ⅜ to ½ inch, for consistent cooking.

Season chicken breasts with salt and black pepper on both sides.

Over medium-high heat, melt coconut oil in a stainless steel skillet until shimmering (shines with flickering light).

Add chicken breasts and sauté until golden brown, about 4 to 6 minutes.

Turn over and brown the other side, about 4 to 6 minutes.

Bake for 6 to 10 minutes until internal temperature is 165 degrees F (74 degrees C).

Spoon tomato sauce on plate; place chicken breast on top of sauce, and spoon additional sauce on top, if desired.

Nutritional breakdown per serving: 231 calories (27.1% from fat); 7 g fat; 39 g protein; 1 g carbohydrate; trace dietary fiber; 99 mg cholesterol; 112 mg sodium.

Tomato Sauce

This sauce freezes well.

MAKES 4 CUPS: ABOUT 16 SERVINGS

⅓ cup virgin coconut oil
2 cups onion, finely chopped
2 pounds tomatoes, vine-ripened, peeled, seeded, and diced
2 garlic cloves, crushed
Bouquet Garni (page 210)
Sea salt or Celtic salt and pepper, to taste

Heat the oil in a saucepan, add the onions, cover and cook for 5 minutes, or until soft and translucent.

Stir in the tomatoes, garlic, Bouquet Garni, and salt and pepper.

Cook for 40 minutes, stirring occasionally, until the mixture is thick.

Discard the Bouquet Garni, season to taste and keep warm.

Nutritional breakdown per serving: 58 calories (68.1% from fat); 5 g fat; 1 g protein; 4 g carbohydrate; 1 g dietary fiber; 0 mg cholesterol; 5 mg sodium.

MISCELLANEOUS RECIPES

Homemade Coconut Milk

This is amazingly easy to make and incredibly delicious.

MAKES ABOUT 1 CUP

1½ cups water
⅞ cup dry unsweetened finely grated coconut

In a medium-size kettle, heat the water, but do not bring it to a boil.

Place the coconut in a blender and add 1 cup of the hot water. Blend for 2 to 3 minutes.

Place a colander in a bowl and line the colander with 4 thicknesses of cheesecloth.

Pour the blended coconut mixture into the cheesecloth and twist to extract the milk, allowing the milk to drip into the bowl.

Return the coconut pulp to the blender and add the remaining ½ cup of hot water. Blend for 1 to 2 minutes, strain and press through the cheesecloth into the bowl.

Nutritional breakdown per serving: 307 calories (58.7% from fat); 21 g fat; 2 g protein; 31 g carbohydrate; 3 g dietary fiber; 0 mg cholesterol; 178 mg sodium.

Almond Milk

Homemade almond milk is much healthier than the commercially packaged almond milk and it's surprisingly easy to make.

Makes 2 cups: 2–4 servings

1 cup ground almonds
2 cups boiling water

Combine almonds and water. Steep for 5 minutes, stirring occasionally.

Sieve the mixture to remove coarse grains or (preferably) blend mixture in electric blender until grains are absorbed.

Nutritional breakdown per serving: 191 calories (71% from fat); 74 g fat; 9 g protein; 7 g carbohydrate; 2 g dietary fiber; 0 mg cholesterol; 7 mg sodium.

Virgin Coconut Oil Mayonnaise

One taste of homemade mayonnaise made with coconut milk will leave the commercial mayonnaise sitting on the grocery store shelf.

MAKES ABOUT 1½ CUPS: ABOUT 12 SERVINGS

1 whole egg
2 egg yolks
1 tablespoon Dijon mustard
1 tablespoon fresh lemon juice
½ teaspoon sea salt or Celtic salt
¼ teaspoon white pepper
½ cup virgin coconut oil, melted if solid
½ cup extra-virgin olive oil

Put the eggs, Dijon mustard, lemon juice, salt, and pepper into a food processor or blender: Then with the processor or blender running on low speed, start adding the oils *very* slowly. Start out with drops and then work up to about a ¹⁄₁₆-inch stream. It should take about 2 minutes to add the oil.

Continue blending until there is no free-standing oil.

Nutritional breakdown per serving: 175 calories (97.1% from fat); 19 g fat; 1 g protein; trace carbohydrate; trace dietary fiber; 51 mg cholesterol; 110 mg sodium.

Aioli (Garlic Mayonnaise)

Use as a dip, sandwich spread, or sauce for fish and chicken.

MAKES 1¼ CUPS

1 large egg yolk
3 garlic cloves, minced
White pepper, to taste
½ cup virgin coconut oil, melted if solid

½ cup extra virgin olive oil
2½ teaspoons fresh lemon juice, or to taste

In a blender or food processor, blend egg yolk, garlic, and pepper on high until smooth. With motor running, gradually drizzle in oils very slowly until creamy and thickened. Start out with drops and then work up to about a ¹⁄₁₆-inch stream. It should take about 2 minutes to add the oil. Add lemon juice and blend well until there is no free-standing oil.

Store covered in refrigerator.

Nutritional breakdown per serving: 99 calories (98.5% from fat); 11 g fat; trace protein; carbohydrate <2 g; trace dietary fiber; 11 mg cholesterol; trace sodium.

Asian Pesto

This pesto goes nicely with grilled fish, chicken, or vegetables.

MAKES 1 CUP: ABOUT 8 SERVINGS

1 cup fresh mint leaves, loosely packed
1 cup fresh cilantro leaves, loosely packed
1 cup fresh basil leaves, loosely packed
¼ cup virgin coconut oil, melted if solid
¼ cup walnuts, chopped
2 tablespoons fresh lime juice
2 garlic cloves, minced
Black pepper, freshly ground

In a blender or food processor, puree all ingredients.
Taste and adjust seasonings.
Store covered in refrigerator until ready to serve. Warm slowly over low heat.

Nutritional breakdown per serving: 91 calories (86.6% from fat); 9 g fat; 1 g protein; 2 g carbohydrate; 1 g dietary fiber; 0 mg cholesterol; 5 mg sodium.

Bouquet Garni

This packet of herbs adds wonderful flavor to any stock or sauce.

SERVES 12

3 leek leaves
1 sprig fresh thyme
4 sprigs fresh parsley
1 bay leaf

Rinse leek leaves; arrange herbs in a spray with leek leaves on the outside. Tie securely with twine, leaving a long tail for easy removal from sauce or stock.

Nutritional breakdown per serving: 0 calories (0% calories from fat); 0 g fat; 0 g protein; 0 g carbohydrate; 0 g dietary fiber; 0 mg cholesterol; 0 mg sodium.

Turkey or Beef Roll-Ups

These roll-ups make a nice snack or a great lunch item when combined with a salad.

SERVES 1 TO 2

2 to 3 slices turkey breast or prime rib or tenderloin
2 to 3 teaspoons soft goat cheese
1 to 2 teaspoons grated zucchini, or several sprigs watercress

Lay the slices of turkey or beef flat on a cutting board.
Spread a thin layer of goat cheese over each slice.
Sprinkle the grated zucchini over the cheese or place sprigs of watercress over the cheese, in the center.
Roll the turkey or beef slices. The end should stick out with a bit

of goat cheese spread at the edges. Eat like a "sandwich" or cut the roll into 1- to 2-inch pieces and serve as an appetizer.

Nutritional breakdown per serving (based on sliced turkey breast): 35 calories (13.5% from fat); >2 g fat; 7 g protein; trace carbohydrate; trace dietary fiber; 13 mg cholesterol; 451 mg sodium.

Coconut Treats

These little treats are a great way to get more coconut oil into your diet and satisfy your need for a sweet fix at the same time.

Serves 1: Makes 1 large treat or 2–3 small ones

1 tablespoon coconut oil, melted or softened if making one large treat; do not melt if forming into balls, just soften
1 to 2 teaspoons ground flax seeds
½ teaspoon pure vanilla extract
¼ to ½ teaspoon stevia or other healthy low-carb sweetener (sweeten to taste)
¼ teaspoon almond extract
⅛ teaspoon sea salt or Celtic salt
Dash of cinnamon
Dash of nutmeg
⅛ cup chopped nuts (almonds or pecans are good) (optional)
2 to 3 teaspoons unsweetened coconut flakes; 4 to 5 teaspoons if rolling in coconut flakes

Mix oil and seasonings. If shaping treats into 1-inch balls, add ½ of the nuts and coconut flakes to the oil mixture and shape it into 1-inch balls. Then roll the balls in the other ½ of the chopped nuts and coconut flakes. Freeze for at least five minutes.

For an alternative shape, you can mix *all* the ingredients, then flatten and shape the mixture into one large macaroon and freeze it in a small bowl. (The ingredients freeze in about 5 minutes.) The coconut treat will pop right out of the bowl and you can eat it like a cookie.

Nutritional breakdown per serving: 125 calories (76.9% from fat); 11 g fat; 3 g protein; 4 g carbohydrate; 2 g dietary fiber; 0 mg cholesterol; 237 mg sodium.

Chapter 7/Phase II

Cleansing—A Weight Loss Advantage

I have observed that when elimination of waste and toxins is increased, weight loss is greatly facilitated. Many people have said cleansing helped them lose weight when nothing else worked. Individuals have also found that adding cleansing programs to their weight loss regimen has improved their health—sometimes dramatically. And, an added bonus is that cleansing often contributes to a more youthful appearance—something many people don't experience on many other weight loss programs.

Certain herbs are especially helpful for weight loss and cleansing. They are a suggested, but optional, part of a cleansing protocol.

HOW THE CLEANSING PROGRAM WORKS

Combine the cleansing protocols for Phase II with the diet and menu plan of Phase III or continue with Phase I, as desired. I recommend that as you cleanse, you don't eat a lot of animal protein. I also recommend that you eat some raw vegetables with each meal.

What follows is a four-step cleansing program that gets results. Signs that your cleanse has been successful include weight loss; loss of wrinkles; healthier skin, hair, and nails; better digestion; increased

I have found over many years of research that because of my thyroid dysfunction, my colon, liver, and gallbladder needed to be cleansed. I recently read about the cleansing diets from Cherie Calbom's book [*The Juice Lady's Guide to Juicing for Health*], and about how the congestion of these organs can make us gain weight. No matter what you try to do to lose weight, until you've cleansed your body, you may not see the weight loss results you want.

I started trying "the cleanses" and I now do not feel so bloated and have lost some weight around my midsection. Cherie recommends the colon first, then the liver, then the gallbladder, and then the kidneys. Things start "clicking and working together" when we remove the toxins. I have not done a full cleanse yet, but so far the results have been good.

—*April*

energy; improved health, a better outlook on life; and a stronger immune system.

Step 1 focuses on colon cleansing (which you may want to continue for four to six weeks if you've never cleansed your intestinal tract before), Step 2 on liver cleansing, Step 3 on gallbladder cleansing, and Step 4 on the kidney flush.

Starting with the first week, you should notice that elimination is greatly improved; you should also drop a couple of pounds. You'll be amazed at the results you'll see as you move on to liver cleansing, gallbladder cleansing, which are closely related, and then to kidney cleansing. Phase II is the rejuvenation phase—the one that produces positive life-changing results that actually show up on your face as well as your waistline.

When you've finished the cleanses you'll undoubtedly get lots of questions and comments about how you're looking and about what you've been doing that's making you look younger, healthier, and trimmer.

FLUSH AWAY THE CELLULITE

It's not just another fat. Simply put, *cellulite* is that lumpy, bumpy or-ange peel–looking skin, which is irregular fat deposits that are found mostly on the thighs, hips, and buttocks. Most of us aren't very happy about these lumps and dimples. Dimples look great on smil-ing young faces, but they don't look so great on thighs.

Infuriatingly, many dieters find that no matter how hard they work at weight loss, exercise, and strict diet, this stuff sticks to the thighs like caramel on an apple—even when they've dropped a size or two.

Because it's quite different from your garden-variety kind of pudge, cellulite has to be attacked in a unique way. Cellulite is asso-ciated with poorly functioning blood vessels, constipation, poor lymphatic drainage, and toxicity.

First off, if blood vessels are weak and sluggish, toxins will accu-mulate quickly, making it difficult for the body to burn fat in the af-fected areas. Essentially, this fat is trapped within connective tissues and the affected area is full of fluid, toxins, lymph, and waste.[1]

Overdoing it on sugar, refined salt (sodium chloride), caffeine, al-cohol, tobacco, unhealthy fats and oils, and refined carbohydrates taxes the lymphatic and circulatory systems. This makes it much harder for the body to eliminate waste—and far easier for cellulite to form. Some experts believe it is toxins that cause this fat to become trapped and held in one spot in the first place.

A diet of refined, high-carbohydrate foods, especially sweets, alcohol, junk foods, and unhealthy oils are tops among the factors that contribute to a sluggish metabolism, and especially a poor-functioning liver. This leads to a buildup of toxins and waste, which can trigger the onset of cellulite. A sluggish, poor-functioning colon causes constipation, which is thought to contribute to cellulite be-cause this condition causes wastes and toxins to be absorbed back into the system rather than being purged.

You can rub, massage, and wrap this fat in seaweed every day of your life, but it's not going to disappear unless you cleanse your body, especially your colon and liver, and improve your circulation and metabolism, get your lymph moving, and nourish your body from within. One particular exercise machine known as a lymphasizer (swing machine), is particularly helpful. (See Resources.) Also, as you boost your metabolism, your circulatory and lymphatic systems will work better, and you'll increase your chances of shifting the bulges.[2]

This kind of fat cannot be eradicated just by eating healthy foods or by exercise. Though creams, lotions, or lymphatic drainage massage may help a little, they will not wipe away the lumps and dimples. Changing your diet and detoxifying your body is key to getting rid of cellulite. You've got to flush out the toxins—plain and simple. "The main processes to follow are those that detoxify rather than [just] promise weight loss," says Shonagh Walker, author of *Cellulite: Not Just a Fancy Name for Fat.*[3]

It's also important to nourish and condition the areas affected with cellulite, strengthen blood vessels and tissues, and step up restricted circulation. Removing toxins and nourishing blood vessels and surrounding tissues make it possible for the body to use fat for energy.

The four-step cleansing program of Phase II, along with exercise, should help you immensely in your fight against the unsightly lumps and bumps. Your thighs don't have to look like a pitted golf ball any longer, and you can be trimmer *and sleeker.*

Numerous testimonies, reports, articles, and book reviews offer firsthand personal experience that says this program works! I can also testify to the fact that it works. I had very noticeable cellulite in my early thirties. Now—after years of cleansing, eating a healthy low-carb diet, and regular exercise—it's virtually gone.

COLON CLEANSING

One of the causes of weight gain and nagging health problems is the formation and buildup of intestinal toxins. Once one truly understands that one of the greatest challenges our body faces is the removal of wastes and toxins, it is difficult to underestimate the importance of cleansing and proper elimination.

CONSTIPATION: A BIG DETERRENT TO WEIGHT LOSS

Constipation refers to the difficulty or infrequency in passing stools due to a sluggish bowel. Constipation can undermine the whole body, affecting digestion, preventing a clearing of toxins, lowering energy levels, and preventing absorption of nutrients. Proper elimination is necessary to avoid a buildup of toxins.

If you want to lose weight efficiently, you need to correct constipation. Poor diet is a major contributor to a sluggish bowel as is poor liver function, parasites, *Candida albicans,* and low thyroid function. Food allergies and sensitivities can also be a contributor as well as dairy products and refined grain products. Stress can also adversely affect the colon. When stressed, the nervous system becomes enzyme deficient, saliva flow decreases, lactic acid accumulates, and digestion is impaired. The treatment of constipation includes adequate fiber, plenty of water, sufficient vitamin C and magnesium, improvement in thyroid health, exercise, and *C. albicans* and parasite cleansing, along with colon and liver cleansing. Drinking fresh vegetable juices can be very helpful as well, since they supply a good source of soluble fiber.

I have observed that when people cleanse the intestinal tract (which includes the colon), constipation is greatly alleviated and weight loss comes much easier and faster.

If you want to lose weight as efficiently as possible and reshape your body, it is absolutely crucial to cleanse the colon (actually the entire intestinal tract) and create an environment for more rapid and successful weight loss results.

Colon cleansing is one of *the most* important steps—and usually the most overlooked—when people attempt to lose weight, reshape the body, flatten the abdomen, and improve digestion and elimination. The problem is that the body cannot properly digest and eliminate some of the foods and substances we ingest. These substances become waste material that can lodge or get stuck in the lining of the intestinal tract in the form of old fecal matter and mucus. People can end up carrying around pounds of this matter that has built up over time, mostly in the colon.

Confounding the body's need for the normal two to three bowel movements per day, this buildup of material interferes with optimal nutrient absorption from our foods and supplements.

Combining colon cleansing with The Coconut Diet can help you trim your waistline faster and more completely. A stomach that protrudes may not be just from fat; it can also be the result of intestinal waste buildup. When the entire intestinal tract is cleansed, the stomach often flattens. The colon can also function better, eliminating wastes quicker, which greatly facilitates weight loss. And nutrient absorption is improved and the body is better fed. As a result, cravings often diminish or disappear, making it easier to stick with the weight loss program.

THE COLON CLEANSE PROGRAM

During the colon cleanse you will continue eating the low-carb, coconut diet, choosing from either Phase I or Phase III recipes. You will incorporate more raw foods and fresh vegetable juices into your diet, along with less animal protein. You are encouraged to eat lighter, smaller portions. Make sure you also drink plenty of water to assist in the cleansing process.

Stick with the Colon Cleanse as long as it takes to complete the job. If you have never tried a colon cleanse, it will probably take four to six weeks to complete the cleansing process. It is rare that the colon can be cleansed in just one week the first time. If you have completed colon cleanses in the past on a regular basis, then one or two weeks will probably work well.

Menu Plan

Upon Rising
7:00 a.m. Fiber Shake

Breakfast
8:00 a.m. Choose from the breakfast recipes and add some raw food such as sliced tomatoes or avocado

9:00 a.m. Probiotic

9:30 a.m. Herbal cleanse formula

10:00 a.m. Fresh vegetable juice such as The Colon Cleanse Juice Cocktail or V-8 juice

11:00 a.m. Fiber Shake

Lunch
12:00 Noon Choose a lunch entrée that incorporates raw vegetables such as one of the main course salads

1:00 p.m. Herbal tea or sparkling water with lemon

1:30 p.m. Herbal cleanse formula

2:00 p.m. Black cherry juice and water

3:00 p.m. Fiber Shake

4:30 p.m. Herbal cleanse formula

Dinner
6:00 p.m. Choose from the dinner entrées and make sure you have some raw vegetables with dinner such as a salad, sliced tomatoes, or vegetable sticks

8:00 p.m. Herbal tea and probiotic

Colon Cleanse Recipes and Products

The colon-cleanse products recommended include psyllium fiber or flax fiber, bentonite clay, and cleansing herbs. You can eat two to three meals a day while cleansing, but they should be light and healthy. You should also include some raw food with each meal.

Fiber Shake

Mix psyllium or flax fiber and bentonite clay together in 8 ounces of water and shake well. Add a teaspoon of pure cranberry or black cherry juice extract to the fiber shake for better flavor and added nutrients (available at health food stores).

The Colon Cleanse Juice Cocktail

1 green apple such as pippin or Granny Smith (only in Phase III or IV) or 1 cucumber, peeled if not organic
1 handful spinach, washed
1 handful parsley, washed
1 stalk celery, rinsed
¼ medium lemon, peeled

Cut the apple or cucumber in half or the size that will fit your juicer feed tube. Bunch up the spinach and parsley and push through the juicer with the apple or cucumber, celery, and lemon.

Black Cherry Juice and Water

Black cherry juice is excellent for cleansing the colon. Unsweetened organic black cherry juice concentrate is available at most health food stores. (A good brand is by Dynamic Health.) Mix 1 to 2 teaspoons in an 8-ounce glass of purified water.

PROBIOTICS

As you cleanse, it is very important to restore the healthy intestinal flora (bacteria) in the gut by taking what is known as a *probiotic* (beneficial bacteria) formula. Often, the body's beneficial bacteria has been depleted by the use of antibiotics, other medications, and years of poor eating habits. Probiotics also restores healthful bacteria after cleansing. Proper bacteria are essential for a strong immune system; assimilation of vitamins, proteins, fats, and carbohydrates; the manufacture of B vitamins, vitamin K, and amino acids; and to keep yeasts such as *Candida albicans* and parasites under control. (For recommendations, see Resources.) Depending on the formula you choose as your probiotic, you may need to take probiotics more or less often than is recommended on our menu schedule.

COLONICS

Colon hydrotherapy, which is popularly known as a *colonic,* entails flushing the colon with water usually by a professional colonic therapist. Colon hydrotherapy is a safe, effective method of removing waste from the large intestine, without the use of drugs. Intestinal waste is softened and loosened by introducing pure, filtered, and temperature-regulated water into the colon, which results in evacuation of waste. A colonic or two per week during the four to six weeks of colon cleansing is particularly helpful to remove excess waste. It can also be helpful in facilitating weight loss.

If you're thinking, "No way would I consider this," it might be of interest to know that some of the most glamorous people we watch in the media have taken advantage of this health practice. It has been reported that Princess Diana was an avid fan of colonics.[4] It's rumored that numerous Hollywood stars take advantage of colonics. The reason partakers range from royalty to Hollywood stars to everyday people is that colonics help to reduce bloating and gas, flatten protruding tummies, facilitate weight loss, improve colon health, and beautify the skin. I have combined colonics with juice fasting and intestinal herbal cleansing several times a year for more than 14 years, and I have on more than one occasion experienced a two-pound weight loss after a colonic. It is recommended that you have one or two colonics per week while doing a colon cleanse.

Toxins can build up on the intestinal wall just like plaque builds up on teeth. Can you imagine never having your teeth cleaned? Well,

> I am almost through with my 30-day general cleanse and about a week ago I finally started feeling better. I began doing about 1½ miles on my Gazelle again. The last time I got on my Gazelle I could only do a mile before becoming so tired that I didn't think I could continue. I am still taking the coconut oil and I finally dropped below 177 pounds—a mark I've been fighting [for a while]. Progress is slow, but I'm starting to feel the benefits of my changes.
>
> —*Tammie*

most people couldn't imagine that, but many people go through life never having their colon cleaned. Colon irrigation hydrates the colon and assists in the removal of built-up fecal matter, mucus, and toxins.[5]

Although it might be disconcerting to the very shy, most practitioners will immediately make you feel relaxed, at ease, and safe. However, make sure the center you choose is clean and uses disposable hoses and tubes.

People who get colonics usually rave about the effects they experience such as improved colon health, flatter tummies, a clearing of the whites of their eyes, improvement in skin health, and a luminescence to their skin. If you cannot find a colon therapist in your area, enemas are the next best thing.

LIVER CLEANSING

The liver performs hundreds of jobs every day that are crucial to life and health. Some of its functions influence weight loss. They include:

- Regulating carbohydrate metabolism, which controls blood sugar
- Regulating protein metabolism, which produces proteins that transport substances such as fat and hormones

- Burning fat for fuel, as well as making cholesterol and fat and storing it
- Regulating hormonal metabolism, especially converting T4 to T3 (thyroid hormones); T4 goes mostly to the liver, where it is converted to T3
- Detoxifying internal toxins and environmental toxins

To lose weight most efficiently, the liver-cleansing week is a must! The liver holds a key to efficient metabolism, weight control, bowel health, and detoxification. The liver is the major fat-burning organ in the body. Cleansing your liver should promote weight loss; you should begin burning fat more efficiently.

When you eat high-carbohydrate foods regularly, your liver makes fat and stores it. This can lead to "fatty liver," which is a buildup of fat in the liver. This can also be associated with toxic exposure and alcohol and caffeine consumption. Statistics show that by the age of 38 the average American experiences a 65 percent drop in liver function due to congestion from toxic buildup. Diabetes and obesity may also contribute to a fatty liver, which in turn leads to inflammation, cell death, and fibrosis (formation of fibrous tissue).[6]

Scientists and physicians are learning that insulin controls a lot of what goes on in the liver, and the liver is a primary organ that can become insulin resistant (see chapter 2 on carbohydrates and insulin resistance).

The liver also stores toxins in fat cells. The more toxins it stores, the more the liver functions are compromised. The liver can become congested just like the colon. When the liver is congested, excretion of bile is inhibited, and a person will be prone to constipation. As toxins linger in the gut too long, they will be absorbed back into the bloodstream. Toxins circulating in the system can cause water retention in certain areas of the body, especially the thighs, hips, and arms. We notice these unsightly collections as lumpy, orange peel–looking skin known as cellulite. A cleansed, well-functioning liver can greatly facilitate the loss of cellulite. (For more information on cellulite, see page 215.)

You may have a number of signs of liver dysfunction, even though all your liver-function blood tests appear normal. The tests used to determine liver function are not designed to show mild dysfunction, but rather liver damage. Symptoms of liver dysfunction include:

- Poor digestion, bloating, gas, weight gain, and constipation
- Irritable bowel syndrome
- Coated tongue or bad breath in the morning
- Mood changes, depression, "foggy" brain
- Allergic conditions such as hay fever, hives, skin rashes, asthma
- Headaches: migraines, tension headaches, hormonal headaches, cluster headaches
- Fluid retention/high blood pressure
- Hypoglycemia/blood sugar instability
- Inability to tolerate fatty foods, nausea, abdominal pains
- Fatigue, chronic fatigue syndrome

On this diet, your liver should give a big sigh of relief and go on about its job of regulating metabolism and burning fat. When the liver is functioning well, weight loss should be greatly facilitated and occur naturally and without excessive effort.

THE 7-DAY LIVER CLEANSE

For seven days, you will follow this menu plan and utilize the low-carbohydrate recipes from the recipe section of Phase I or III for your meals. Additional recipes follow the 7-day plan.

Menu Plan

Upon Rising
7:00 a.m. or upon rising drink 1 cup hot water with the juice of ¼ lemon and a dash of cayenne pepper

7:15 a.m. Beet juice cocktail (juice cucumber, carrots, a beet with greens, celery, parsley, ginger root, and lemon)

Breakfast

8:00 a.m. Choose any breakfast suggestion from the breakfast recipes and include some raw food
Supplement: 1 to 2 capsules of the herb milk thistle or liver-cleansing herbs. (See Resources.)
9:00 a.m. 1 to 2 teaspoons Beet Salad (page 226)
10:30 a.m. Ginger or echinacea herbal tea
11:00 a.m. 1 to 2 teaspoons Beet Salad

Lunch

12:00 Noon Choose any entrée from the Lunch section and include some raw food
Supplement: 1 to 2 capsules of the herb milk thistle or liver-cleansing herbs
1:15 p.m. 1 to 2 teaspoons Beet Salad
3:00 p.m. Green Drink (page 226): Juice as many greens as you like. Start with a base of cucumber, celery, and lemon. To that add parsley, kale, spinach, sprouts, or any other greens. If juice is not possible, mix powdered greens in water.
3:30 p.m. 1 to 2 teaspoons Beet Salad
4:30 p.m. A cup of herbal tea (optional)
5:15 p.m. 1 to 2 teaspoons Beet Salad

Dinner

6:00 p.m. Carrot Salad with Lemon–Olive Oil Dressing (page 226)
One cup Potassium-Rich Vegetable Broth (page 227)
Main course salad or entrée of choice from the Dinner entrées*
Supplement: 1 to 2 capsules milk thistle or liver-cleansing herbs
7:15 p.m. 1 to 2 teaspoons Beet Salad
8:30 p.m. Chamomile or peppermint herbal tea

Avoid eating after 7:30 p.m. to give your liver a chance to do its work of cleansing while you sleep.

*Include artichokes often; they are very liver supportive

Liver Cleansing Recipes and Products

Beet Salad

2 tablespoons extra-virgin, cold-pressed olive oil
Juice of ½ lemon
1 cup raw beets, finely grated or very finely chopped

Whisk the olive oil and lemon juice together and mix with the beets. Eat one to two teaspoons of this salad every two hours during the day for seven days.

Carrot Salad with Lemon–Olive Oil Dressing

Place 1 cup of finely shredded carrots, or carrot pulp leftover from juicing, in a bowl. If shredding the carrots, they should be a mushy consistency; use a food processor or fine grater. (It's easiest to use the carrot pulp.) For the dressing, combine 1 tablespoon extra-virgin, cold-pressed olive oil with a tablespoon of fresh lemon juice and a dash of cinnamon (optional). Whisk together. You may add more dressing, but not less. Pour the dressing over the shredded carrots (or carrot pulp) and mix well.

Green Drink

Preferably in the afternoon, drink 10 ounces freshly juiced green vegetables—cucumber, parsley, spinach, kale, celery, or any other green herb or vegetable. Add fresh lemon juice and/or freshly juiced ginger root to pep up the flavor. Fresh mint also makes a nice addition with cucumber and other milder-tasting greens.

Potassium-Rich Vegetable Broth

This vegetable broth provides important nutrients, especially minerals, your body needs during the cleansing process. Eat 1 to 2 cups of the broth daily.

MAKES ABOUT 6 SERVINGS

**2 to 3 cups chopped fresh green beans (string beans) (frozen is
  acceptable when fresh is not available)
2 to 3 cups chopped zucchini
2 to 3 stalks celery
Purified water, for steaming
1 to 3 tablespoons chopped parsley
1 tablespoon chopped garlic
Seasonings and herbs, to taste
Coconut oil (optional)**

Steam the green beans, zucchini, and celery over purified water until soft, but still green and not mushy.

Place the cooked vegetables, plus the raw parsley and garlic, in a blender and puree until smooth.

Add a bit of the steaming water, as needed, but keep the broth fairly thick.

Season to taste with minced ginger, cayenne, vegetable seasoning, or herbs of your choice.

Add coconut oil to the broth, if desired.

Milk Thistle (Silymarin)

Take one or two capsules of the herb milk thistle with each meal. Milk thistle contains some of the most potent liver-cleansing compounds known. Silymarin, the most active ingredient in milk thistle, enhances liver function. It also has excellent antioxidant properties that help prevent damage to the liver. Or, look for a liver-cleansing herbal combination that has milk thistle in it.

LIVER-CLEANSING HERBS

There are various cleansing herbal formulas for detoxifying the liver, improving liver function, increasing bile flow, reducing swelling, and purifying the blood. They can be partnered with herbs used to strengthen the liver's glandular and organ functions. Such herbs help remove fat deposits associated with consuming too many unhealthy fats, damaged fats, sugar, and alcohol, as well as chemical exposure. They also help increase lecithin production, which keeps cholesterol more soluble. These formulas are best used following the colon cleanse. For more information, see Resources.

GALLBLADDER CLEANSING

The liver and gallbladder are interconnected and work together. What affects one will affect the other—both positively and negatively. One of the primary routes of eliminating toxins is through the bile. Bile is made in the liver and concentrated in the gallbladder. It becomes a carrier substance by which to expel many toxins from the body. Impaired bile flow results in stools that may be hard and difficult to pass and contribute to toxic buildup.

Weight gain can also be a sign of a congested gallbladder. Signals of gallbladder congestion include fatty food intolerance (trouble digesting fats), belching, bloating, headache, and strong appetite.

> I had my gallbladder removed 20 years ago, so I have to support my liver and elimination. If my body gets too "toxic," I will find myself awake with a racing mind, even though I'm not under any other kind of stress. Good cleansing can help one sleep.
>
> —*Monique*

Intense pain in the abdomen that radiates to the upper back can be an indication of gallstones. Ultrasound provides a definitive diagnosis. Approximately 20 percent of the women and 8 percent of the men over 40 in the United States experience gallstones. Each year this leads to surgery to remove more than 300,000 gallbladders.

It is important to note that during weight loss, concentration of cholesterol in the bile actually increases, setting the stage for gallstones. Secretion of all bile components is reduced during weight loss, but secretion of bile acids decreases more than cholesterol. One function of bile acids is to keep cholesterol in solution. This setup greatly increases the risk of gallstone formation or acceleration of stone growth.

Once weight is stabilized, bile acid output returns to normal and the cholesterol production remains low. The overall effect is an improvement in bile solubility with weight loss. This is one good reason for a gallbladder cleanse while on a weight loss program. Anyone losing more than one pound per week should follow the general guidelines for gallstone prevention (page 135).

It is especially important to eat good fats during an intense weight loss program—only extra virgin olive oil and virgin coconut oil with small amounts of butter. Coconut oil is an easy-to-digest fat due to its concentration of medium chain triglycerides, making it a good dietary choice while cleansing.

THE 7-DAY GALLBLADDER FLUSH

The 7-Day Gallbladder Flush is easy to incorporate, even into a busy lifestyle. It can greatly improve the function of this secondary organ of elimination and thereby facilitate weight loss. Digestion of fats as well as digestion in general should improve. Following is a menu plan for this week:

Menu Plan

Upon Rising
Hot water, lemon and cayenne pepper
Olive oil and lemon juice
Follow with a cup of herbal peppermint tea

Breakfast
Breakfast of your choice from breakfast recipe section (page 153)
  with some raw food such as sliced tomatoes or avocado
9:00 a.m. 1 to 2 teaspoons Beet Salad (page 226)
10:00 a.m. Fresh vegetable juice such as the Gallbladder Cleansing Cocktail (page 231), V-8 juice, or fresh pear juice (pear is
  cleansing for the gallbladder)
10:30 a.m. 8 ounces of water with lemon (⅛ to ¼ lemon)*
11:00 a.m. 1 to 2 teaspoons Beet Salad
11:30 a.m. Ginger or echinacea herbal tea

Lunch
12:00 noon Lunch entrée from lunch recipes (page 162). Choose
  a main course salad as often as possible.
1:00 p.m. 1 to 2 teaspoons Beet Salad
2:00 p.m. Fresh vegetable juice
3:00 p.m. 1 to 2 teaspoons Beet Salad
4:00 p.m. 8 ounces of water with lemon (⅛ to ¼ lemon)
5:00 p.m. 1 to 2 teaspoons Beet Salad

Dinner
Fresh vegetable juice
6:00 p.m. Dinner entrée from dinner recipes (page 183); make
  sure you have a salad or raw veggies
Supplement: LipotropicFormula (page 232)
7:00 p.m. 1 to 2 teaspoons Beet Salad
8:00 p.m. Herbal tea such as chamomile or peppermint

*Lemon is very cleansing for the gallbladder

Gallbladder-Cleansing Recipes and Products

Hot Water, Lemon Juice, and Cayenne Pepper

Lemon and cayenne are excellent liver and gallbladder cleansers.

Upon rising, squeeze ¼ of a fresh lemon in a cup (8 ounces) of warm to hot purified water and add a small dash of cayenne pepper. Stir together.

Olive Oil and Lemon Juice

In the morning upon rising mix 2 tablespoons extra virgin olive oil and 1 to 2 tablespoons fresh lemon juice in 4 to 6 ounces purified water or juice.

Mix vigorously; down quickly!

Drink this mixture for seven days.

Gallbladder Cleansing Cocktail

1 handful parsley, washed
4 medium carrots, scrubbed well, green tops removed, ends
trimmed
2 stalks celery with leaves, washed, ends trimmed
½ lemon, peeled

Bunch up the parsley and push it through the juicer feed tube with the carrots, celery, and lemon.

Stir the juice and pour into a glass.

Drink as soon as possible to maximize the nutritional value, store in the refrigerator, covered, or take in a thermos.

Additional Glasses of Fresh Vegetable Juice

• Carrot, beet, and cucumber juice
• Carrot, celery, and endive or kale juice
• Carrot, beet, and coconut milk
• Carrot and spinach

Note: If you are sugar sensitive (hypoglycemic or diabetic) and react to carrots or beets, then use cucumber and more greens, and flavor with lemon juice or ginger.

Beet Salad

MAKES ABOUT 1 CUP

1 cup raw beets, finely grated or chopped
2 tablespoons extra virgin, cold-pressed olive oil
Juice of ½ lemon

Whisk the olive oil and lemon juice together and mix with the grated beet.

Eat 1 to 2 teaspoons of this salad every two hours during an eight-hour period for seven days.

LIPOTROPIC FORMULA

A lipotropic formula includes choline, methionine, taurine, HCL betaine, folic acid, and vitamin B6. This combination of nutrients helps remove fat from the liver and increases bile solubility. Take as directed. (See Resources.)

KIDNEY CLEANSING

When we cleanse, it is as important to include the kidneys, too. During cleansing, the kidneys must process more toxic substances than normal. A number of herbs are beneficial in strengthening and toning the kidneys. They help increase urine flow, reduce inflammation, and remove uric acid and other crystalline formations. The 7-Day Kidney Flush that follows contains natural food and herbal diuretics that not only support the kidneys but also facilitate water weight loss.

The 7-Day Kidney Flush Menu Plan

Upon rising
Drink 1 cup of herbal tea such as agrimony, marshmallow, juniper, or buchu. (These can be found at health food stores.) These diuretic herbs will help rid the body of excess water and they benefit the urinary tract as well.

Fresh juice such as Kidney Tonic or Cranberry Water (page 234)

Breakfast
8:00 a.m. Breakfast of your choice from breakfast recipes (page 153); add some raw food such as sliced tomatoes or avocado

10:00 a.m. Nettles Tea (and kidney herbal supplement, as desired) (See Resources.)

11:00 a.m. Cranberry Water

Lunch
12:00 noon Lunch entrée from salads (page 162), soups and stews (page 177), or vegetable dishes (page 180); strive for a main course salad as often as possible

2:00 p.m. Cranberry water (and kidney herbal supplement, as desired)

4:00 p.m. Cranberry Water

Dinner
6:00 p.m. Dinner entrée from dinner recipes (page 183) with a salad or raw veggies

8:00 p.m. Herbal tea (and herbal supplement, as desired)

Kidney Cleansing Recipes and Products

Cranberry Water

Mix 1 to 2 teaspoons unsweetened cranberry concentrate, which can be purchased at health food stores. Add a little stevia or other low-carb sweetener to sweeten, if desired. (Dynamic Health makes an excellent organic cranberry concentrate.)

Nettles Tea

The herb nettles is used traditionally for kidney cleansing and support; it helps eliminate uric acid. Drink 1 cup of this tea each day. In addition, take an herbal supplement that will help detoxify the kidneys. (See Resources.)

Kidney Tonic

1 cucumber, peeled if not organic
Handful parsley
1 stalk celery
¼ lemon, peeled or handful of mint
½-inch piece ginger root

Cut the cucumber in half and juice.

Bunch up the parsley and juice followed by the celery, lemon or mint, and ginger. (Parsley and celery are kidney tonic juices.)

Note: Cucumber, watermelon, cantaloupe with seeds, asparagus, lemon, kiwifruit, and parsley are all considered natural diuretics.

KIDNEY CLEANSE HERBAL SUPPLEMENTS

You may also wish to take an herbal supplement that will help detoxify the kidneys. (See Resources.)

Chapter 8/Phase III

Introducing Healthy Carbs

After three weeks on Phase I, you can switch to Phase III of The Coconut Diet, which includes limited amounts of whole grains, fruits, and starchy vegetables. If you choose to incorporate Phase II—Cleansing—you can follow either Phase I or Phase III of the meal plan during the cleanse weeks, depending on what works best for your weight loss and cleansing needs. When you have completed the cleansing program, you will stay with Phase III until you have lost the weight you desire.

During Phase III gradually introduce some of the healthiest carbs—whole grains, fruits, and some starchy vegetables such as acorn squash, corn, and sweet potatoes—into the weekly menu plan. Of course, no matter which phase you're in, continue to incorporate coconut oil into your diet.

I recommend that you start reintroducing these foods with no more than three to four whole grain servings, three to four fruit servings, and two to three starchy vegetable servings per week, as desired. You may eat less of these servings, but not more unless you find you're still losing weight. The menu plan is a guideline, but you should adjust it accordingly. This will slow your weight loss, but you should still lose, on average, two pounds a week. However, if you have any of the conditions discussed in chapters 4 and 5 such as hypothyroid, *Candida albicans*, fibromyalgia, hypoglycemia, or digestive problems, then you should avoid Phase III foods until your condition is corrected. Follow the dietary program outlined for your condition in chapter 4 or 5.

As you develop more lean tissue (which burns more calories even at a resting heart rate), balance blood sugar, and correct insulin resistance, you can add a few additional servings of the healthy carbs per week, providing you continue to lose the weight you desire. You will continue to avoid all refined carbs.

There may be times when you indulge in too many carbs or foods that are off the list—at parties, special events, or on vacation. Or you may experience times of emotional stress that trigger binge eating, and as a result, you may put on a few pounds. The most important point to remember at such times is that you don't want to throw caution to the wind by telling yourself you've "blown it" and now you may as well eat whatever you want. (If you find yourself overeating, binge eating, or choosing the wrong foods for emotional reasons, see pages 94–96.) This is the time to get right back on the program. At this point I recommend that you go back to Phase I. You may want to incorporate the 1-Day Vegetable Juice Cleanse (page 132) as a weight loss kick-start, which will also help cleanse your body.

FOODS YOU CAN REINTRODUCE

Dairy
Milk
Plain yogurt

Fruit

Apples	Grapes
Apricots	Kiwifruit
Blackberries	Loganberries
Blueberries	Mangoes
Cantaloupe	Oranges
Cherries	Papaya
Grapefruit	Peaches

Pears   Raspberries
Plums   Strawberries

Grains
Amaranth
Barley (thought of as a grain, actually a cereal grass)
Buckwheat
Buckwheat groats (kasha)
Cornmeal (coarse polenta)
Kamut
Millet
Oats (rolled, steel-cut)
Quinoa
Rice (all whole varieties); no white rice
Spelt
Wheat (whole only)

Vegetables
Corn
Squash: acorn, buttercup, butternut, hubbard
Sweet potatoes
Yams

Miscellaneous
Carob
Unsweetened chocolate (cocoa); only if you do not have hypo-
    glycemia or impaired thyroid or adrenal function

FOODS TO AVOID

Dairy
Frozen yogurt
Ice cream
Soymilk
Yogurt: fruit flavors and sweetened

Fruit
Bananas
Canned fruit
Dried fruit such as dates, prunes, and raisins
Fruit juice (with the exception of black cherry and cranberry concentrate; small amounts only)
Pineapple
Watermelon

Grains/breads
All refined grains as found in:

Bagels
Bread: refined wheat, white
Breadsticks
Breakfast cereals: all cereals except whole grain cereals
Buns/dinner rolls
Crackers (except dehydrated seed crackers)
Instant oatmeal
Matzo
Muffins (except low-sugar, whole grain)
Pasta (except whole grain)
Pizza dough
Rice, white
Rice cakes

Potatoes
Idaho
New white
Red skinned

Snack Foods
All snack foods such as:

Cheese snack foods
Corn chips
Potato chips

Soy snack foods
Tortilla chips

Sweeteners
Artificial sweeteners
Brown rice syrup
Fructose
Honey
Jam/Jellies
Malt barley syrup
Maple syrup
Sugar of all types
Syrups (including high-fructose corn syrup)

BASIC PREPARATION TECHNIQUES

Following are guidelines for the cooking techniques and procedures for whole grains and beans used most frequently in Phase III recipes.

Cooking brown rice: Place 1 cup of rice in a heavy pan. Cover with water and swish around. Drain rice in a fine wire strainer. Return rice to pan and cover with 1½ to 2 cups water or vegetable stock and add ½ teaspoon sea salt or Celtic salt, if using. Bring to a rolling boil. Reduce heat, cover, and cook over low heat for about 45 minutes. (Add more liquid if the rice becomes too dry.) Avoid removing the lid or stirring until the last 5 minutes. Uncover for the last 5 minutes and cook over very low heat, shaking the pot occasionally. When the rice is done, fluff with a fork.

Cooking dried beans: Place the beans in a colander and rinse under running water, culling any bad ones. Place the beans in a bowl or pan with water to cover by 2 or 3 inches and let them soak for 8 to 10 hours; doing this overnight is usually easiest. Drain and rinse the beans. Put the beans in a large kettle or Dutch oven with 4 cups of water for every 1 cup of beans. Bring the water to a boil, then reduce the heat, cover, and simmer until the beans are tender, about

1½ hours. Stir the beans occasionally as they cook and add more water if necessary to keep them from sticking to the bottom of the pot. Do not add salt to the beans until they are done (adding salt during cooking will toughen them).

An alternative to soaking the beans for hours is to place the beans in a heavy pot with water to cover by 2 inches and bring to a boil for 1 minute; remove from heat, cover, and let soak for 1 to 2 hours and then cook according to the directions above. Or use canned beans.

For added flavor, add 1 onion studded with 3 or 4 whole cloves to the pot while cooking. Discard the onion and cloves before using the beans.

Cooking grains—For all grains except amaranth, cornmeal, and teff: Wash the grains if desired. (Quinoa is the only grain that *must* be washed to remove the saponin, a bitter coating.) In a heavy saucepan with a tight-fitting lid, bring the recommended quantity of liquid to a boil. Add the grain and a pinch of salt, if desired. Reduce the heat, cover, and simmer for the specified time (see Cooking Times for Grains, opposite). Do not stir. If grains need more liquid before they have finished cooking, add a bit of boiling water and continue to cook.

For amaranth, cornmeal, and teff: Combine the grain with water in a saucepan and bring to boil. Reduce the heat and simmer, uncovered, for the specified amount of time, stirring occasionally.

Cooking Times for Grains

GRAIN (1 CUP DRY MEASURE)	LIQUID	COOKING TIME	YIELD
Amaranth	2 cups	30 minutes	2 cups
Barley	2 cups	60 minutes	4 cups
Buckwheat	1½–1¾ cups	20 minutes	3½ cups
Bulgur (parboiled, cracked wheat)	1½ cups	15 minutes	2½ cups
Cornmeal (course polenta)	3–4 cups	25 minutes	2 cups
Cracked wheat	1½ cups	25 minutes	2½ cups
Kamut	1½ cups	1½ hours	2 cups
Millet	2–2½ cups	15–20 minutes	4 cups
Oats rolled	2 cups	10 minutes	3 cups
steel-cut	2 cups	15–20 minutes	3 cups
whole groats	2 cups	60 minutes	3 cups
Quinoa	2 cups	10–15 minutes	2–2½ cups
Rice (all variations)	1¼–1½ cups	45–50 minutes	2–2½ cups
Spelt	1¼–1½ cups	1–1¼ hours	2 cups
Triticale	1¾ cups	2 hours	2½ cups
Wheat berries	1½ cups	2 hours	2½ cups
Wild rice	1¾ cups	55–60 minutes	2½ cups

THE 1-WEEK MENU PLAN

DAY 1

Breakfast
Green or herbal tea with lemon
1 to 2 soft-boiled eggs
1 slice turkey or beef bacon

Mid-Morning Break
Cup of herbal tea with lemon
6 to 10 macadamia nuts

Lunch
Apple-Pecan Turkey Salad with Creamy Vinaigrette (page 249)

Mid-Afternoon Snack
½ cup plain yogurt with 1 tablespoon chopped nuts, and a pinch of
    cinnamon
Sparkling mineral water with a slice of lemon

Dinner
Thai Coconut Salmon Over Wild Rice (page 259)
Steamed broccoli
Sliced cucumbers and onions with rice vinegar or Asian Citrus
    Dressing (page 250)
1 Feather Light Coconut Macaroon (page 271)

DAY 2

Breakfast
Green or herbal tea with lemon
6 to 8 ounces vegetable juice, preferably fresh
Basic Scrambled Eggs (page 154)
1 to 2 slices turkey bacon

Mid-Morning Break
1 to 2 Turkey or Beef Roll-Ups (page 210)

Lunch
Spinach salad with pine nuts and avocado and Asian Citrus Dressing (page 250)

Mid-Afternoon Break
Sparkling mineral water with a slice of lemon
12 raw or toasted almonds

Dinner
Broiled fish
Quinoa Millet Croquettes (page 254)
Steamed zucchini and onion
Crispy green salad with Coconut Ranch Dressing (page 252)

DAY 3

Breakfast
Green or herbal tea with lemon
6 to 8 ounces vegetable juice, preferably fresh
Eggs Benedict with Turkey Ham (page 159)
Jicama Pancakes (page 247)

Mid-Morning Break
Green or herbal tea with lemon
12 raw or toasted almonds

Lunch
Sliced turkey on green salad with Coconut Ranch Dressing (page 252)

Mid-Afternoon Break
Sparkling mineral water with a slice of lemon
Vegetable sticks

Dinner
Chicken Curry (page 260) over wild rice
Steamed vegetables of choice
Sliced tomatoes and cucumbers with rice vinegar

DAY 4

Breakfast
Green or herbal tea with lemon
6 to 8 ounces vegetable juice, preferably fresh
Bowl of millet or amaranth (see page 240 for grain cooking instructions) with Almond Milk (page 207), Coconut Milk (page 206), or dairy

Mid-Morning Break
Green or herbal tea with lemon
12 raw or toasted almonds

Lunch
Soup and salad with one piece of Cornbread (page 256)

Mid-Afternoon Break
Sparkling mineral water with a slice of lemon
Vegetable sticks

Dinner
Indian Coconut Vegetable Curry (page 261)
Wild rice or brown basmati rice
Small cucumber salad with Yogurt Sauce with Lemon (page 264)

DAY 5

Breakfast
Green or herbal tea with lemon
6 to 8 ounces vegetable juice, preferably fresh
1 poached egg

1 slice Bread Machine Bread with Coconut Oil (page 257), toasted and spread with butter or virgin coconut oil or Ezekiel bread (available at most natural markets and health food stores)

Mid-Morning Break
Green or herbal tea with lemon
½ cup fresh berries: blueberries, blackberries, or raspberries. (Frozen can be substituted when fresh is not available.)

Lunch
Spinach Avocado Salad with Citrus-Balsamic Vinaigrette (page 251)

Mid-Afternoon Break
Sparkling mineral water with a slice of lemon
Sliced tomatoes with balsamic vinegar and extra-virgin olive oil or vegetable sticks

Dinner
Quinoa-Stuffed Acorn Squash (page 262)
Steamed vegetables of choice
Cucumber salad with Yogurt Sauce with Mint and Garlic (page 268)

DAY 6

Breakfast
Green or herbal tea with lemon
6 to 8 ounces vegetable juice, preferably fresh
Steamed Eggs (page 248)
1 to 2 slices of turkey or beef bacon

Mid-Morning Break
Green or herbal tea with lemon
12 raw or toasted almonds

Lunch
Bowl of soup with ½ Coconut Carrot Muffin (page 258)

Mid-Afternoon Break
Sparkling mineral water with a slice of lemon
Vegetable sticks

Dinner
Baked or broiled fish with Yogurt Sauce with Curry (page 265)
Brown Basmati Coconut Pilaf (page 255)
Green salad with Citrus-Balsamic Vinaigrette (page 251)
Dessert: Coconut Pineapple Sorbet (page 272)

DAY 7

Breakfast
Green or herbal tea with lemon
6 to 8 ounces vegetable juice, preferably fresh
Basic Cheese Omelet (page 157)
1 slice turkey or beef bacon

Mid-Morning Break
Green or herbal tea with lemon
10 to 12 raw or toasted almonds

Lunch
Spinach Avocado Salad with Citrus-Balsamic Vinaigrette (page 251)

Mid-Afternoon Break
Sparkling mineral water with a slice of lemon
Hummus (garbanzo dip; can be found premade at most grocers)
    and vegetables

Dinner
Baked chicken with Béchamel Sauce made with almond milk,
    coconut milk, or dairy (pages 268–270)
Steamed vegetables of choice
Green salad with dressing of choice

BREAKFAST RECIPES

Jicama Pancakes

SERVES 4

1 medium jicama, peeled
¼ cup red onion, finely chopped
¼ cup whole grain flour
1 teaspoon sea salt or Celtic salt
1 large egg, beaten
2 tablespoons virgin coconut oil
Dollop sour cream or yogurt

Shred or grate jicama (using large holes of grater), combine with chopped or grated red onion.

Sprinkle with flour and salt and stir to combine.

Add beaten egg and stir to combine.

Heat coconut oil in medium skillet over medium-high heat until shimmering.

Drop quarter-cup dollops of jicama mixture into skillet, flattening into pancake shape, cook until golden brown, about 2 to 4 minutes.

Turn and brown the other side, about 2 to 4 minutes.

Serve with sour cream or plain yogurt.

Nutritional breakdown per serving: 167 calories (42.8% from fat); 8 g fat; 4 g protein; 21 g carbohydrate; 9 g dietary fiber; 47 mg cholesterol; 491 mg sodium.

Steamed Eggs

Soft and creamy like custard, this simple dish tastes quite luxurious.

Serves 2

4 eggs
Filtered water, as needed
1 tablespoon virgin coconut oil
1 cup sliced mushrooms
2 scallions, sliced
2 teaspoons soy sauce, or to taste

Break the eggs into a measuring cup. Measure an equal amount of water.

Beat together the eggs and water. Then pour the eggs into an ovenproof bowl.

Place a steaming rack in the bottom of a pan that is large enough to hold the bowl of eggs. Do not allow the bowl to touch the bottom of the pan. (It can be as simple as a few chopsticks placed in the bottom of the pan.) Place the bowl of eggs on the rack and add enough water to reach about halfway up the side of the bowl.

Cover the pan with aluminum foil and bring the water to a boil. Reduce the heat to simmer, cover, and cook until the eggs are firm.

While the eggs are cooking, heat the coconut oil in a small pan. Add the sliced mushrooms and sauté for about 2 minutes. Add the scallions and sauté for a minute or two more.

When the eggs are done, top them with the mushroom-scallion mixture and sprinkle with soy sauce to taste.

Nutritional breakdown per serving: 203 calories (69% from fat); 16 g fat; 4 g protein; 12 g carbohydrate; 4 g dietary fiber; 374 mg cholesterol; 458 mg sodium.

SALADS

Apple-Pecan Turkey Salad

SERVES 2

6 ounces sliced turkey breast, cut into bite-size strips
½ cup chopped Granny Smith or pippin apple
½ cup chopped celery
10 toasted pecans, chopped
3 to 4 cups mixed salad greens of choice
¼ to ⅓ cup Creamy Vinaigrette (below)

In a medium salad bowl, place all ingredients except the salad dressing.

Spoon the dressing over the salad a little at a time, while tossing.

Nutritional breakdown per serving (does not include vinaigrette): 223 calories (41.8% calories from fat); 11 g fat; 23 g protein; 11 g carbohydrate; 5 g dietary fiber; 35 mg cholesterol; 1,265 mg sodium.

Creamy Vinaigrette

MAKES ABOUT ½ CUP: SERVES 4

¼ cup red wine vinegar
1 tablespoon finely chopped chives or scallions
½ teaspoon sea salt or Celtic salt
¼ teaspoon or equivalent healthy low-carb sweetener
1 clove garlic, crushed
Pinch savory or oregano
Pinch cayenne pepper
2 tablespoons Virgin Coconut Oil Mayonnaise (page 208) or
    mayonnaise of choice

In a small bowl, whisk together the vinegar, chives or scallions, salt, sweetener, garlic, savory or oregano, and cayenne.

Add the mayonnaise and whisk until well blended. Refrigerate until ready to use.

Nutritional breakdown per serving: 33 calories (63.6% from fat); 2 g fat; >2 g protein; 3 g carbohydrate; trace g dietary fiber; 2 mg cholesterol; 288 mg sodium.

Asian Citrus Dressing

This dressing is delicious on spinach salad or mixed green salads.

MAKES 1 CUP: ABOUT 8 SERVINGS

1 garlic clove, minced
1 teaspoon fresh ginger, peeled and minced
2 tablespoons scallions, minced
2 tablespoons fresh lime juice
2 tablespoons fresh orange juice
1 tablespoon rice wine vinegar
2 teaspoons low-sodium soy sauce
¼ cup virgin coconut oil, melted if solid
¼ cup sesame oil
1 dash cayenne pepper

In a blender or food processor, combine all ingredients and blend until smooth.

Taste and adjust seasonings.

Store covered in refrigerator. Bring to room temperature before using.

Nutritional breakdown per serving: 124 calories (95.5% calories from fat); 14 g fat; trace protein; 1 g carbohydrate; trace dietary fiber; 0 mg cholesterol; 50 mg sodium.

Spinach Avocado Salad with Citrus-Balsamic Vinaigrette

This salad is nice garnished with pistachio nuts.

SERVES 4

½ pound fresh spinach, washed and stemmed
1 cup avocado, cubed
½ cup Citrus-Balsamic Vinaigrette (below)
Pistachio nuts for garnish

Wash spinach and remove tough stems. Spin dry in salad spinner or pat dry with paper towels. Tear into bite-size pieces and place in large bowl.

Add cubed avocado to bowl of spinach.

Drizzle with Citrus-Balsamic Vinaigrette and toss to coat.

Garnish with nuts and serve immediately.

Nutritional breakdown per serving: 195 calories (84.0% from fat); 19 g fat; 2 g protein; 6 g carbohydrate; 3 g dietary fiber; 0 mg cholesterol; 205 mg sodium.

Citrus-Balsamic Vinaigrette

Orange juice combines nicely with balsamic vinegar to make a delicious variation to the basic balsamic vinaigrette.

MAKES 1 CUP: ABOUT 16 SERVINGS

2 tablespoons balsamic vinegar
½ teaspoon sea salt or Celtic salt, to taste
¼ teaspoon freshly ground black pepper, to taste
3 tablespoons orange juice (fresh is best)
1 tablespoon Dijon mustard
1 garlic large clove, juiced or pressed
¼ cup virgin coconut oil, melted if solid
¼ cup extra-virgin olive oil

Combine all ingredients except the oils and mix well.
Combine coconut oil and olive oil, stirring until liquid.
While whisking, drizzle in oil very slowly in a steady stream.

Nutritional breakdown per serving: 62 calories (96.0% from fat); 7 g fat; trace protein; 1 g carbohydrate; trace dietary fiber; 0 mg cholesterol; 78 mg sodium.

Coconut Ranch Dressing

Here's a great ranch dressing that makes an equally delicious dip for veggies.

MAKES 1¼ CUPS: ABOUT 12 SERVINGS

⅓ cup plain yogurt
⅓ cup Virgin Coconut Oil Mayonnaise (page 208) or mayonnaise
  of choice
½ cup buttermilk
2 teaspoons finely grated onion
1 small garlic clove, pressed
Sea salt or Celtic salt and freshly ground black pepper, to taste
1 tablespoon fresh chives, snipped

Whisk the yogurt, mayonnaise, and buttermilk together.
Stir in the onion and garlic.
Season with salt and a generous grinding of pepper, then fold in the chives.
Refrigerate, covered, until ready to use (up to 8 hours).

Nutritional breakdown per serving: 47 calories (82.3% from fat); 4 g fat; 1 g protein; 1 g carbohydrate; trace dietary fiber; 12 mg cholesterol; 40 mg sodium.

SOUPS

Creamy Vegetable Soup

This soup takes just 35 minutes to make but tastes like it has simmered for hours.

SERVES 6

1 large tomato
4 carrots
4 stalks celery
1 tablespoon virgin coconut oil
2 cups chopped onion
1 teaspoon savory
4 to 6 garlic cloves, minced
10 to 15 sun-dried tomato halves, cut into small pieces
2 cups milk (plain almond milk can be substituted)
½ cup whole wheat/brown rice flour
½ teaspoon sea salt or Celtic salt

Cut the tomato into wedges. Cut the greens off the carrots. Juice the tomato, carrots, and celery, and reserve 2½ cups of the combined juice. If you don't have enough juice, add more celery.

Heat the oil in a large, heavy skillet over low heat. Add the onions, savory, and garlic, and sauté, stirring occasionally until the onions are tender.

In a medium-size, heavy saucepan, combine the sun-dried tomatoes, milk, and flour. Bring the mixture to a boil, stirring constantly. Then reduce the heat, cover the saucepan, and simmer, stirring occasionally, until the mixture is very thick and the dried tomato pieces are tender, about 10 minutes.

Add the sun-dried tomato mixture to the sautéed onions in the kettle and stir. Slowly add the combined juice to the kettle, stirring vigorously with a wire whisk to keep the mixture from lumping. (If the milk mixture is very hot when the juice is added, it will not lump.)

Add the salt and stir. Either serve the soup immediately or store in the refrigerator until ready to serve. To reheat, bring it to a boil, reduce the heat, and simmer for 2 to 3 minutes before serving.

Nutritional breakdown per serving: 161 calories (19.7% from fat); 4 g fat; 6 g protein; 28 g carbohydrate; 4 g fiber; 11 mg cholesterol; 398 mg sodium.

GRAIN SIDE DISHES

Quinoa Millet Croquettes

These crispy, mild-flavored croquettes are a delicious accompaniment to vegetable dishes. Serve them plain or with a sauce. For an exotic flavor, try them with the added orange or tangerine peel.

SERVES 3 TO 4

½ cup millet
½ cup quinoa
2 cups filtered water
1 tablespoon tahini (sesame paste)
½ teaspoon sea salt or Celtic salt
2 tablespoons minced sweet onion
2 tablespoon minced parsley
1 teaspoon ground cumin
2 to 3 teaspoons grated or finely minced organic orange or
    tangerine peel (optional)
2 tablespoons virgin coconut oil

Place the millet and the quinoa in a medium-size saucepan. Cover with water, swish it around to wash, and then drain it through a fine wire strainer. Return the grain to the pan. Add 2 cups filtered water. Cover and bring to a boil. Reduce the heat to simmer, and cook over low heat for about 20 minutes, or until the water is completely absorbed.

Let the grain cool until it is comfortable enough to touch. Do not refrigerate it because it will cause the mixture to dry out and not stick together well. Add the remaining ingredients, except for the coconut oil. Mix well and shape by hand into 6 to 8 patties.

Heat the coconut oil in a large skillet and brown the patties on both sides. Serve immediately.

Nutritional breakdown per serving (based on 4 servings): 260 calories (38% from fat); 11 g fat; 35 g carbohydrates; 4 g dietary fiber; 6 g protein; 2 mg cholesterol; 247 mg sodium.

Brown Basmati Coconut Pilaf

When brown rice is cooked like this, every grain is separate.

Serves 3 to 4

1 cup brown basmati rice
2 tablespoons virgin coconut oil
6 cardamom pods
1 teaspoon pink peppercorns
2 teaspoons turmeric
3 tablespoons dry unsweetened finely shredded coconut
½ teaspoon sea salt or Celtic salt
Pinch of saffron
2 cinnamon sticks
2⅓ cups boiling water

Wash the rice and drain it through a wire strainer. Set aside.

In a large skillet that has a lid, heat the coconut oil. Add the cardamom pods, peppercorns, turmeric, and coconut. Stir over medium-high heat until the coconut begins to brown. This will happen quickly; do not burn it.

Add the rice and stir for 1 minute more. Add the salt, saffron, and cinnamon sticks. Pour the boiling water over the rice mixture. Cover immediately and cook over low heat for about 40 minutes, or until all the water is absorbed. Fluff with a fork and serve.

Nutritional breakdown per serving (based on 4 servings): 287 calories (32% from fat); 10 g fat; 5 g protein; 5 g carbohydrate; 5 g dietary fiber; 0 mg cholesterol; 252 mg sodium.

Cornbread

This cornbread is very light, with a crispy crust and faint taste of coconut. Leftover cornbread is good sliced through the middle and frozen. To reheat, brush the cut sides with a little coconut oil and broil until hot and toasty.

MAKES 8 PIECES

1½ cups cornmeal
¼ teaspoon ascorbic acid powder (vitamin C powder)*
2 teaspoons baking powder
1 teaspoon baking soda
¼ to ½ teaspoon sea salt or Celtic salt
¼ cup virgin coconut oil (melted if solid)
3 eggs
¾ cup milk (unflavored rice milk, or organic dairy)
2 tablespoons virgin coconut oil

Preheat oven to 375 degrees F.

In a large bowl, combine the cornmeal, ascorbic acid powder, baking powder, baking soda, and salt. Mix well.

Add the coconut oil and the eggs. Mix again. Add the milk and mix well.

In a 9- or 10-inch cast-iron skillet, melt 2 tablespoons coconut oil. Pour the batter into the skillet and spread it out evenly.

Cook over a large burner, over medium-high heat until the batter in the skillet starts to bubble. Be careful not to burn the bottom.

Transfer the skillet to the top rack of the oven and bake for 15 to 20 minutes or until the cornbread is firm to the touch.

*The ascorbic acid powder is not necessary, but it helps the cornbread to rise.

Nutritional breakdown per serving (analysis with dairy milk): 221 calories (20% from fat); 13 g fat; 5 g protein; 38 g carbohydrate; 22 g dietary fiber; 2 mg cholesterol; 73 mg sodium.

Bread Machine Bread with Coconut Oil

Coconut oil adds a delicious flavor to ordinary whole wheat bread.

MAKES A 1-POUND LOAF: 12 SERVINGS

1 cup filtered water
2 cups whole wheat flour
1 tablespoon dry active yeast
2 tablespoons virgin coconut oil
½ teaspoon sea salt or Celtic salt
¼ cup vital gluten flour*
1 tablespoon pure maple syrup

Place all the ingredients in a bread machine on a whole wheat setting, and let process until done.

*Gluten flour is wheat flour that has some of its starch removed and its protein concentrated, producing flour that is 70 percent gluten. Adding gluten flour to a yeast-bread recipe makes the bread light and spongy.

Nutritional breakdown per serving: 115 calories (23% from fat); 3 g fat; 7 g protein; 16 g carbohydrate; 3 g dietary fiber; 0 mg cholesterol; 98 mg sodium.

Coconut Carrot Muffins

These muffins are light, moist, and not too sweet.

MAKES 12 MUFFINS

1 tablespoon virgin coconut oil, or as needed
1 tablespoon whole wheat pastry flour
2 cups whole wheat pastry flour
½ tablespoon baking powder
1 tablespoon cinnamon
¼ teaspoon nutmeg
¼ teaspoon ascorbic acid powder, optional
1 cup grated carrots
2 eggs
1 teaspoon stevia (Lo Han Guo or birch sugar can be substituted;
  use ¼ cup birch sugar or other sweetener)
3 tablespoons virgin coconut oil
1 cup warm filtered water

Preheat oven to 350 degrees F.

Brush a 12-cup muffin tin with 1 tablespoon coconut oil and sprinkle it with the 1 tablespoon of flour.

In a mixing bowl, combine the 2 cups of flour with the baking powder, cinnamon, nutmeg, and ascorbic acid powder, if desired. Mix well. Add the carrots and mix again.

In another bowl, beat together the eggs, stevia, coconut oil, and warm (not hot) water, then add the flour mixture to the liquid mixture.

Spoon mixture equally within the prepared muffin tins.

Bake for 20 minutes, or until firm and an inserted toothpick comes out clean.

Nutritional breakdown per serving: 136 calories (40% from fat); 6 g fat; 4 g protein; 18 g carbohydrates; 3 g dietary fiber; 31 mg cholesterol; 19 mg sodium.

LUNCH OR DINNER ENTRÉES

Thai Coconut Salmon Over Wild and Brown Rice

This dish adds delicious flavor to salmon. A wild and brown rice bed for the salmon and sauce makes a nice accompaniment, and is useful for soaking up this lovely curry sauce.

SERVES 3 TO 4

1 (13.5-ounce) can coconut milk, regular or lite, or Homemade
   Coconut Milk (page 206)
1 tablespoon red curry paste
¼ to ½ cup fish sauce
1 tablespoon healthy low-carb sweetener; only 1 teaspoon of
   stevia or Lo Han Guo
12 ounces fresh salmon or similar firm-fleshed fish
Several fresh basil leaves (optional)
1 cup cooked brown and wild rice (optional)
2 to 3 bunches spinach, steamed (optional)

In a wok or large skillet, heat coconut milk over medium heat. Add curry paste and stir constantly. Simmer until paste is dissolved. Add fish sauce and sweetener and cook for 1 minute.

Place salmon into the mixture and simmer while spooning mixture over fish. Cook for 8 minutes or until fish is completely done (opaque in center).

Garnish with fresh basil leaves, as desired.

Serve over brown and wild rice or steamed spinach. *Suggestion:* ¼ cup rice per serving.

Nutritional breakdown per serving: 380 calories (69% from fat); 130 g fat; 9 g protein; 11 g carbohydrate; 2 g dietary fiber; 47 mg cholesterol; 189 mg sodium.

Chicken Curry

A medley of steamed vegetables and a wild and brown rice bed for the chicken and sauce make a nice accompaniment, and is useful for soaking up this lovely curry sauce.

SERVES 3 TO 4

3 to 4 tablespoons virgin coconut oil
2 cups chopped onion
2 to 3 green hot peppers (optional)
1 tablespoon freshly minced garlic*
2 teaspoons coriander
1½ teaspoons turmeric
6 to 8 chicken thighs**
¾ (13.5-ounce) can coconut milk
3 tablespoons fresh lemon juice
Sea salt or Celtic salt, to taste (optional)

Heat a heavy pan; add the oil and onions and sauté gently until they are soft and transparent. Don't rush this part. It is very important that the onions be really softened and cooked to a slightly golden color. Only then will they be ready for the spices. This could take as much as 15 to 20 minutes.

Add the peppers. For a little touch of spiciness, seed the peppers (remove the seeds) and chop them up finely. For lots of spiciness, leave the peppers whole with the seeds intact. Now add the minced garlic and spices and sauté for another 3 minutes, stirring constantly.

Pushing the onions aside, add the chicken pieces to the pan and cook to a slightly golden color. Turn them around and cover them with the onion spice mixture.

Stir in the coconut milk, then simmer for at least 45 minutes until the chicken is tender. By cooking this dish slowly for a lengthy period, you ensure that the meat will absorb all the lovely flavors of the spices and the coconut milk.

Add the lemon juice and it's ready to serve. If the lemon is very large and juicy, use only half. Add little, if any, salt to this dish.

*Always use fresh garlic, never garlic salt or garlic powder; it will ruin the taste of the dish!

** It is preferable, and certainly healthier, to use free-range chicken, which is much leaner and tastier than factory-bred chicken.

A dollop of plain yogurt will be cooling, especially if the "hot" version is used. (A dollop is a large tablespoon or two of yogurt.) This is an excellent antidote for spiciness and blends very well with any curry flavor.

Nutritional breakdown per serving: 493 calories (66% from fat); 37 g fat; 24 g protein; 20 g carbohydrate; 4 g dietary fiber; 69 mg cholesterol; 91 mg sodium.

Indian Coconut Vegetable Curry

This deliciously spiced curry tastes like a dish one might enjoy in a favorite Indian restaurant.

SERVES 4 TO 6

**2 cups brown basmati rice
1 medium tomato, cut into chunks
1 onion, coarsely chopped
½ inch slice fresh ginger
3 tablespoons dry unsweetened finely shredded coconut
1 tablespoon curry powder
1 teaspoon cumin
1 teaspoon ground cardamom
1 teaspoon pink peppercorns
2 tablespoons virgin coconut oil
4 medium carrots, sliced
1 small cauliflower, broken in flowerets
1 small eggplant, cubed
1 teaspoon sea salt or Celtic salt
Cayenne pepper, to taste (start with a dash and adjust to taste)**

Wash the rice and place it in a pan with 4 cups of water. Cover and bring the water to a boil. Reduce heat and simmer over medium-low heat for 45 minutes, or until the water is absorbed. While the rice cooks, prepare and cook the vegetable curry.

Place the tomato, onion, and ginger in a blender. For easy blending, make sure to add the tomato first. Blend to a paste.

In a small bowl, combine the coconut, curry powder, cumin, cardamom, and peppercorns.

Heat the coconut oil in a large, heavy kettle and add the coconut spice mixture. Stir over medium-high heat just until the coconut begins to brown. This will happen quickly, so be careful not to burn the coconut.

Add the blended tomato mixture. Stir and cook, uncovered, for about 3 minutes.

Add the vegetables and salt. Stir and cover. Reduce the heat to medium low and cook, stirring occasionally until the vegetables are tender, about 15 minutes or more, depending on the size of the vegetable pieces. Add a dash of cayenne to taste and serve over the brown basmati rice, accompanied by a dish of spicy dahl, as desired. (Dahl is a thick stew or dip made from pulses, which are dried beans, peas, or lentils, with onions and spices.)

Nutritional breakdown per serving (based on 6 servings): 363 calories (19% from fat); 5 g fat; 9 g protein; 67 g carbohydrates; 9 g dietary fiber; 0 mg cholesterol; 57 mg sodium.

Quinoa-Stuffed Acorn Squash

A great dish on a winter night! This could be a main dish with a side salad.

SERVES 4

3 acorn squash, halved and seeded
1 tablespoon virgin coconut oil
½ cup chopped onion

½ cup quinoa, rinsed and drained
1 cup vegetable stock
Sea salt or Celtic salt, to taste
Freshly ground black pepper, to taste
¼ cup toasted almonds, chopped
1 clove garlic, minced
2 tablespoons chopped fresh parsley
4 tablespoons Parmesan cheese

Preheat oven to 350 degrees F.

Arrange squash, cut side down, in a baking pan. Add ½ inch water to the pan and cover with aluminum foil. Bake until squash is tender, 30 to 45 minutes (depending upon the size of the squash). Leave oven on.

While the squash is baking, heat the coconut oil in a skillet over medium heat. Add the onions and cook until tender and starting to appear golden, 8 to 10 minutes. Stir in the quinoa, coat with the coconut oil; and toast lightly. Add the vegetable stock and heat to boiling. Reduce heat, cover, and simmer for approximately 15 minutes.

When the squash is cool enough to handle, scoop out and dice the pulp of two squash halves. Turn the other four halves cut side up and season lightly with salt and pepper. Stir the toasted almonds, garlic, parsley, 2 tablespoons of the cheese and diced squash into the quinoa. Spoon into the squash cavities. Sprinkle the tops with the remaining Parmesan cheese.

Return to oven and bake an additional 15 to 20 minutes until heated through.

Nuritional breakdown per serving: 359 calories (26.8% from fat); 11 g fat; 11 g protein; 59 g carbohydrate; 8 g dietary fiber; 12 mg cholesterol; 546 mg sodium.

SAUCES

Yogurt Sauce with Lemon

This is a great sauce to accompany fish.

MAKES 1¼ CUPS: ABOUT 8 SERVINGS

1 cup plain yogurt
1 teaspoon lemon zest, finely grated
1 tablespoon fresh lemon juice
¼ cup fresh mint or parsley, chopped
Sea salt or Celtic salt and freshly ground black pepper, to taste

Gently drain the liquid from the top of the yogurt before combining with the other ingredients so that the flavors are not diluted.
Combine all of the ingredients in a small bowl.
Refrigerate, covered, until needed.

Nutritional breakdown per serving: 18 calories (3.5% from fat); trace fat; 2 g protein; 3 g carbohydrate; trace dietary fiber; 1 mg cholesterol; 23 mg sodium.

Yogurt Garlic Sauce

For more flavor, make this sauce a day ahead, cover, and chill in the refrigerator.

MAKES 1 CUP: ABOUT 8 SERVINGS

1 teaspoon chopped garlic
½ teaspoon sea salt or Celtic salt
1 cup plain yogurt (preferably whole-milk)
1 tablespoon fresh lemon juice

Mash garlic to a paste with salt using a mortar and pestle (or mince and mash with a heavy knife). Stir together garlic paste, yogurt, and lemon juice.

Nutritional breakdown per serving: 20 calories (44.5% from fat); 1 g fat; 1 g protein; 2 g carbohydrate; trace dietary fiber; 4 mg cholesterol; 132 mg sodium.

Yogurt Sauce with Curry

This fabulous sauce will add an Asian flair to fish or chicken dishes.

MAKES 1⅓ CUPS: ABOUT 12 SERVINGS

¾ cup plain yogurt
2 tablespoons mango chutney
1 teaspoon fresh lime juice, or to taste
½ cup Virgin Coconut Oil Mayonnaise (page 208) or mayonnaise of choice
1 tablespoon curry powder, or to taste
2 tablespoons minced red onion, plus an additional teaspoon for garnish
Sea salt or Celtic salt and freshly ground black pepper, to taste

In a blender or small food processor blend together ½ cup of the yogurt, chutney, and the lime juice until the mixture is smooth. Transfer the mixture to a bowl, and whisk in the remaining ¼ cup yogurt, mayonnaise, curry powder, 2 tablespoons onion, and salt and pepper to taste.

Chill the sauce, covered, for at least 8 hours and up to 3 days.

Transfer the sauce to a serving dish and garnish it with the additional onion.

Nutritional breakdown per serving: 82 calories (88.6% from fat); 8 g fat; 1 g protein; 2 g carbohydrate; trace dietary fiber; 5 mg cholesterol; 102 mg sodium.

Yogurt Sauce with Feta Cheese

This sauce is great drizzled over a salad of fresh mixed greens and can be made 2 days ahead: Cover and refrigerate.

MAKES 1 CUP: ABOUT 8 SERVINGS

3 ounces feta cheese, crumbled
½ cup plain yogurt
2½ tablespoons chopped fresh chives
1½ tablespoons fresh lemon juice
1 teaspoon dried oregano
Sea salt or Celtic salt and freshly ground black pepper, to taste

Using a fork, mash the feta cheese in small bowl.
Mix in remaining ingredients.
Season to taste with salt and pepper.
Let stand 30 minutes to allow flavors to develop. Store in the refrigerator.

Nutritional breakdown per serving: 39 calories (63.2% from fat); 3 g fat; 2 g protein; 2 g carbohydrate; trace dietary fiber; 11 mg cholesterol; 126 mg sodium.

Yogurt Sauce with Lime-Cilantro

This sauce can be prepared 1 hour ahead; cover and chill.

MAKES 3½ CUPS: ABOUT 12 SERVINGS

2 cups plain yogurt (whole-milk is preferable)
1 cup cucumber, peeled, seeded, and diced
1 cup chopped fresh cilantro
2 tablespoons fresh lime juice
Sea salt or Celtic salt and freshly ground pepper, to taste

Blend all ingredients in processor using on/off turns just until cucumber is finely chopped.

Season with salt and pepper and transfer to a small bowl.

Nutritional breakdown per serving: 28 calories (20.5% from fat); 1 g fat; 2 g protein; 3 g carbohydrate; trace dietary fiber; 2 mg cholesterol; 30 mg sodium.

Yogurt Sauce with Mint and Carrots

This sauce is excellent with chicken. Make up to 8 hours ahead and chill.

MAKES 2 CUPS: ABOUT 8 SERVINGS

2 cups plain yogurt (whole-milk is preferable)
2 teaspoons cumin seed
2 medium carrots, finely grated
¼ cup fresh mint leaves, finely chopped
Sea salt or Celtic salt and freshly ground black pepper, to taste

In a sieve set over a bowl, drain yogurt; cover and chill for 2 hours.

In a dry, small heavy skillet toast cumin seeds over moderate heat, shaking skillet frequently, until a shade darker, 2 to 3 minutes. Cool cumin seeds and with a mortar and pestle or in an electric coffee/spice grinder coarsely grind them.

Add carrots to a small bowl and stir in yogurt, cumin, mint, and salt and pepper to taste.

Nutritional breakdown per serving: 48 calories (38.7% from fat); 2 g fat; 2 g protein; 5 g carbohydrate; 1 g dietary fiber; 8 mg cholesterol; 36 mg sodium.

Yogurt Sauce with Mint and Garlic

Make this yogurt sauce up to 1 day ahead, cover and chill. Bring to room temperature before serving.

MAKES 1 CUP: ABOUT 8 SERVINGS

1 cup plain yogurt (whole-milk is preferable)
1 garlic clove, minced
2 tablespoons chopped fresh mint
Sea salt or Celtic salt and freshly ground black pepper, to taste

Drain yogurt in a sieve lined with a double thickness of cheese-cloth at room temperature for 20 minutes.

Stir together with garlic, mint, and salt and pepper to taste.

Nutritional breakdown per serving: 20 calories (44.7% from fat); 1 g fat; 1 g protein; 2 g carbohydrate; trace dietary fiber; 4 mg cholesterol; 15 mg sodium.

Béchamel Sauce with Almond Milk

For a traditional white sauce without the dairy, this béchamel is quite good made with almond milk.

MAKES 3 CUPS: ABOUT 12 SERVINGS

1 tablespoon minced onion
3 tablespoons virgin coconut oil
¼ cup whole grain flour
3 cups Almond Milk (page 207) or premade (plain)
¼ teaspoon sea salt or Celtic salt
White pepper, to taste

In a saucepan, cook the onion in coconut oil over moderately low heat, stirring, until it is softened. Stir in the flour and cook the roux, stirring, for 3 minutes.

Add the milk in a stream, whisking vigorously until the mixture is thick and smooth, add the salt and the white pepper, and simmer the sauce for 10 to 15 minutes, or until it is thickened to the desired consistency.

To prevent a skin from forming, strain the sauce through a fine sieve into a bowl and cover the surface with a buttered round of wax paper.

Nutritional breakdown per serving: 134 calories (72.6% from fat); 12 g fat; 5 g protein; 5 g carbohydrate; 2 g dietary fiber; 0 mg cholesterol; 48 mg sodium.

Béchamel Sauce with Coconut Milk

This traditional white sauce is delicious made with coconut milk and coconut oil.

MAKES 3 CUPS: ABOUT 12 SERVINGS

1 tablespoon minced onion
3 tablespoons virgin coconut oil
¼ cup whole grain flour
3 cups Homemade Coconut Milk (page 206) or canned coconut milk
¼ teaspoon sea salt or Celtic salt
White pepper, to taste

In a saucepan, cook the onion in the coconut oil over moderately low heat, stirring, until it is softened. Stir in the flour and cook the roux, stirring, for 3 minutes.

Add the coconut milk in a stream, whisking vigorously until the mixture is thick and smooth, add the salt and the white pepper, and simmer the sauce for 10 to 15 minutes, or until it is thickened to the desired consistency.

To prevent a skin from forming, strain the sauce through a fine sieve into a bowl and cover the surface with a buttered round of wax paper.

Nutritional breakdown per serving: 176 calories (85.2% from fat); 18 g fat; 2 g protein; 5 g carbohydrate; 2 g dietary fiber; 0 mg cholesterol; 54 mg sodium.

Béchamel Sauce with Dairy

This is the traditional version of béchamel.

MAKES 3 CUPS: ABOUT 12 SERVINGS

1 tablespoon minced onion
3 tablespoons virgin coconut oil
¼ cup whole grain flour
3 cups whole milk
¼ teaspoon sea salt or Celtic salt
White pepper, to taste

In a saucepan, cook the onion in the coconut oil over moderately low heat, stirring, until it is softened. Stir in the flour and cook the roux, stirring, for 3 minutes.

Add the milk in a stream, whisking vigorously until the mixture is thick and smooth, add the salt and the white pepper, and simmer the sauce for 10 to 15 minutes, or until it is thickened to the desired consistency.

To prevent a skin from forming, strain the sauce through a fine sieve into a bowl and cover the surface with a buttered round of wax paper.

Nutritional breakdown per serving: 76 calories (63.5% from fat); 5 g fat; 2 g protein; 5 g carbohydrate; trace dietary fiber; 8 mg cholesterol; 74 mg sodium.

DESSERTS AND TREATS

Feather Light Coconut Macaroons

These baked goods made with whole wheat flour are anything but heavy.

MAKES ABOUT 18 COOKIES

1 tablespoon virgin coconut oil, as needed
1 tablespoon whole wheat pastry flour, as needed
3 egg whites
1 teaspoon vanilla
1 teaspoon stevia or other healthy low-carb sweetener; less, or
    more to taste, depending on choice of sweetener
½ cup dry unsweetened finely shredded coconut
⅓ cup whole wheat pastry flour
½ teaspoon baking soda
1 teaspoon lemon juice
2 tablespoons pure maple syrup

Preheat oven to 300 degrees F. Grease a cookie sheet with 1 table-spoon coconut oil and sprinkle it with 1 tablespoon flour.

Beat the egg whites until they are stiff enough to stand in peaks. Beat in the vanilla and the stevia. Set aside.

In a separate bowl, combine the coconut (⅓ cup), flour, and baking soda. Mix well, then add the lemon juice and the maple syrup. Mix again.

Carefully fold the egg whites into the coconut mixture and drop it by the spoonful onto the prepared cookie sheet.

Bake for 20 to 25 minutes or until golden, then turn off the oven, remove the cookies from the cookie sheet, and transfer them to a baker's rack (or the racks of the oven). Let them set in the warm oven for another 20 minutes.

Nutritional breakdown per cookie: 31 calories (12% from fat); 2 g fat; 1 g protein; 4 g carbohydrates; trace dietary fiber; 0 mg cholesterol; 80 mg sodium.

Coconut Pineapple Sorbet

This impressive dessert is so delicious it is hard to believe that it does not contain sugar. To make it you will need a blender, a juicer, and an ice cream maker.

SERVES 6

1 recipe Homemade Coconut Milk (page 206) or equal amount canned coconut milk (1 cup)
1 fresh pineapple, peeled and cut into spears (or 2 cups commercial juice)
¼ teaspoon stevia or other healthy low-carb sweetener, or to taste
1 teaspoon pure vanilla extract
2 tablespoons virgin coconut oil

Follow the recipe for coconut milk, and place the coconut milk in a large measuring cup.

Run the pineapple through a juicer. Reserve all of the juice and ⅓ cup of the pulp. (If you do not juice fresh pineapple, blend canned pineapple [drained] in the blender to create pulp. This will not be as good, but can be substituted.)

Place enough of the pineapple juice in the cup with the coconut milk to make 3 cups liquid. If you do not have enough, add a little filtered water.

Place the liquid mixture in a blender with the remaining ingredients, except for the pulp, and blend. Pour the mixture into an ice cream maker, add the pulp, and process according to directions until frozen. Enjoy!

Nutritional breakdown per serving: 197 calories (72% from fat); 17 g fat; 1 g protein; 13 g carbohydrates; 1 g dietary fiber; 0 mg cholesterol; 8 mg sodium.

Chapter 9/Phase IV

Maintaining Your Healthy Weight

When you have reached your goal weight, you are ready for Phase IV. This phase of the plan is designed to help you maintain your ideal weight. By now your biochemistry should have improved considerably, and you should be at a place where cravings for sweets, breads, and starches have virtually disappeared. You are ready to eat a wide variety of healthy foods that will help you stay trim for the rest of your life.

In Phase III you probably tried a number of different grains and vegetables and some new recipes. The Meal Plan and recipes in Phase IV will help you continue to choose hale and hearty meals and snacks that taste great. The foods you'll avoid from this point on are the ones that not only pack on the weight, but also contribute to poor health. At this point, there is only a list of foods to avoid as much as you possibly can. If you do indulge in foods on the avoid list or overindulge in carbohydrate-rich foods once in while, you can always return to Phase I, II, or III until you lose the pounds you gained. If you binge on unhealthy foods while on vacation or during an emotionally stressful time, then you should cleanse your body, incorporating the Colon and Liver Cleanses of Phase II. And, keep in mind that it is always a good idea to cleanse your body on a quarterly basis to achieve and maintain radiant, vibrant health.

By following these steps, you should be able to maintain your desired weight for life. Best of all, you have embarked on an excellent disease-prevention program. This will help you avoid heart disease, cancer, diabetes, stroke, and other debilitating conditions. You're on your way to *living a life of abundant physical and mental energy combined with a positive outlook on life.* That's the definition of vitality—and it can be yours by choice!

FOODS TO AVOID

Animal Proteins
Beef
> All fatty cuts that include: brisket, liver, liverwurst, rib eye steak, ribs

Pork
> In general is not the healthiest, but especially avoid: bacon, honey-baked ham

Poultry: processed poultry products

Beverages
Alcohol: beer, liquor, wine
Anything with artificial flavors or sweeteners
Canned, bottled, or frozen fruit juice (any fruit juice that has been pasteurized; vitamins and enzymes are destroyed with high heat, leaving mainly sugar and water.)
Chocolate drinks/sweetened cocoa
Coffee
Diet sodas and all soda pop
Sports drinks

Dairy
Ice cream
Processed cheeses
Sweetened yogurt

Fats
Commercial salad dressings and mayonnaise made with any of the oils in the following list:

Margarine
Polyunsaturated oils: canola, corn, safflower, soybean, sunflower

Grains
All refined wheat and white flour products which include:

Bagels	English muffins
Biscuits	Muffins
Bread	Oatmeal (instant)
Bread sticks	Pancakes
Breakfast pastries	Pasta
Buns	Pizza dough
Cereal bars	Rolls
Cereals	Stuffing
Crackers	Tortillas
Doughnuts	Waffles

Snack Foods
Cheese snacks
Chips: corn, potato, tortilla
Microwave popcorn; hydrogenated and partially hydrogenated oils are harmful
Pretzels
Soy crisps and snacks

Sweets (especially commercially prepared)
It is best to make your own treats with our recommended sweeteners and healthy ingredients.

Barbecue sauce with sugar
Desserts: brownies, cakes, candy, cookies, ice cream, mousse, pies, pudding, sugar-sweetened gelatin (Jell-O)
Energy bars with refined sweeteners
Jams
Jellies

Ketchup
All sugars and artificial sweeteners
Syrup (artificial syrups; choose pure maple syrup)

THE 1-WEEK MENU PLAN

DAY 1

Breakfast
Green or herbal tea with lemon
Cooked whole-grain cereal such as amaranth or oatmeal with fresh
  berries and almond milk, dairy milk, or cream

Mid-Morning Break
Herbal tea with lemon
20 raw or toasted almonds

Lunch
Southwestern Black Bean Soup (page 285)
Small mixed green salad with oil and vinegar dressing or
  homemade vinaigrette

Mid-Afternoon Snack
1 celery stalk stuffed with almond butter, cut into six pieces
Sparkling mineral water with a slice of lemon

Dinner
Garlic-Parmesan Halibut (page 295)
Butternut Squash, Sage, and Blue Cheese Gratin (page 290) or
  baked sweet potato
Steamed green beans with sliced almonds
Mixed green salad with vinaigrette dressing (pages 172–176)

DAY 2

Breakfast
Green or herbal tea with lemon
Chef's Cheezy Eggs (page 281)
Fresh fruit cup or sliced tomatoes sprinkled with herbs

Mid-Morning Break
Pippin or Granny Smith apple

Lunch
Cream of 4-Mushroom Soup (page 286)
Green salad with Citrus-Balsamic Vinaigrette (page 283)

Mid-Afternoon Break
Hummus (garbanzo dip, available premade at most grocers) with
   vegetable sticks

Dinner
Grilled fish with lemon and herbs
Butternut Squash, Sage and Blue Cheese Gratin (page 290)
Crispy green salad with your favorite vinaigrette

DAY 3

Breakfast
Green or herbal tea with lemon
6 to 8 ounces vegetable juice, preferably fresh
Basic Cheese Omelet (page 157)
1 to 2 strips turkey or beef bacon

Mid-Morning Break
Turkey or Beef Roll-Up (page 210)

Lunch
Curried Chicken Grape Salad (page 284)

Mid-Afternoon Break
1 Coconut Treat (page 211) or Feather Light Coconut Macaroon
(page 271)

Dinner
Baked chicken with Béchamel Sauce (almond, coconut, or dairy)
(pages 268–270)
Caramelized Onion and Squash Gratin (page 291)
Caesar salad

DAY 4

Breakfast
Green or herbal tea with lemon slices
Basic Scrambled Eggs (page 154)
1 to 2 strips turkey or beef bacon

Mid-Morning Break
Herbal tea
3 dehydrated crackers spread with virgin coconut oil or almond
butter

Lunch
Split pea or lentil soup
Caesar salad

Mid-Afternoon Break
1 Coconut Treat (page 211)

Dinner
Chicken Curry (page 260)
Blend of wild and brown rice
Crispy green salad with Coconut Ranch Dressing (page 252)

DAY 5

Breakfast
Green or herbal tea with lemon slices
Unbelievable Baked Eggs (page 162)
1 to 2 strips turkey or beef bacon

Mid-Morning Break
½ pear

Lunch
Grilled salmon Caesar salad
1 Coconut Carrot Muffin (page 258)

Mid-Afternoon Break
½ apple

Dinner
Grilled steak and mushrooms
Steamed broccoli
Sliced tomatoes with buffalo mozzarella and fresh basil with balsamic vinegar and olive oil

DAY 6

Breakfast
Green or herbal tea with lemon slices
Smoothie of your choice

Mid-Morning Break
Herbal tea
1 hard-boiled egg

Lunch
Cream of 4-Mushroom Soup (page 286)
Spinach salad with Citrus-Balsamic Vinaigrette (page 283)

Mid-Afternoon Break
Veggie sticks with Aioli (page 208)

Dinner
Thai Green Vegetable Curry (page 294)
Blend of brown and wild rice
Green salad with Citrus Balsamic Vinaigrette (page 283)

DAY 7

Breakfast
Green or herbal tea with lemon slices
Avocado and Cream Cheese Frittata (page 282)
Crispy green salad or spinach salad

Mid-Morning Break
6 to 8 ounces vegetable juice, preferably fresh

Lunch
Carrot-Pineapple Slaw (page 289)
Tomato-Basil Soup (page 288)

Mid-Afternoon Break
Sparkling mineral water with a slice of lemon
3 to 4 dehydrated crackers or rye crisps spread with almond butter
    or coconut oil

Dinner
Roasted Squash with Poblano Pepper and Jack Cheese Quesadillas
    with Chipotle Lime Sour Cream (page 293)
Cup of Gazpacho (page 177)

BREAKFAST RECIPES

Chef's Cheezy Eggs

A delicious entrée for that special breakfast or brunch.

SERVES 2

4 large eggs
3 ounces cream cheese, cut into ½-inch cubes
¼ cup Parmesan cheese, grated
Black pepper, freshly ground, to taste
1½ tablespoons virgin coconut oil
1 garlic clove, minced

In a small bowl, beat eggs with cream cheese cubes, Parmesan cheese, and black pepper. Set aside.

In a nonstick skillet, melt coconut oil over medium-high heat. When coconut oil is hot and bubbly, add garlic and sauté about a half minute.

Pour egg mixture into skillet. Stir and fold gently until cream cheese is melted and eggs are cooked to preferred doneness. Serve immediately.

Nutritional breakdown per serving: 415 calories (79.4% from fat); 37 g fat; 8 g protein; 3 g carbohydrate; trace dietary fiber; 429 mg cholesterol; 423 mg sodium.

Avocado and Cream Cheese Frittata

This makes a fabulous dish for a weekend brunch. A crisp green salad is a good complement.

SERVES 2

4 large eggs
2 tablespoons heavy cream
2 teaspoons fresh herbs such as parsley, basil, thyme, oregano, minced
Black pepper, freshly ground
Dash cayenne pepper
2 tablespoons virgin coconut oil

Filling

1 small red onion, diced
1 garlic clove, minced
1 tablespoon virgin coconut oil
3 tablespoons cream cheese, cut into ½-inch cubes

Garnish

1 large avocado, peeled and sliced.

Preheat broiler.

In a medium bowl, whisk eggs, cream, fresh herbs, black pepper, and cayenne pepper. Set aside.

In a nonstick skillet, melt the 1 tablespoon of coconut oil over medium-high heat. When oil is hot and bubbly, add onion and garlic and sauté until softened, about 5 minutes. Set aside.

In a medium-size oven-proof skillet, melt the 2 tablespoons of coconut oil over medium-high heat. When oil is hot and bubbly, add egg mixture. As eggs cook, lift edges to allow uncooked egg to seep underneath. When bottom is set but top is still moist, place cream cheese cubes and onion mixture over eggs and place under broiler.

Broil 1 to 2 minutes, checking frequently, until top is golden and puffed up.

Top with sliced avocado. Serve immediately.

Nutritional breakdown per serving: 630 calories (79.7% from fat); 58 g fat; 16 g protein; 17 g carbohydrate; 4 g dietary fiber; 418 mg cholesterol; 195 mg sodium.

SALADS AND DRESSINGS

Citrus-Balsamic Vinaigrette

This is a delicious variation of a basic balsamic vinaigrette.

MAKES 1 CUP: ABOUT 16 SERVINGS

2 tablespoons balsamic vinegar
½ teaspoon sea salt or Celtic salt, to taste
¼ teaspoon black pepper freshly ground, to taste
3 tablespoons fresh orange juice
1 tablespoon Dijon mustard
1 large garlic clove, juiced
¼ cup virgin coconut oil, melted if solid
¼ cup extra-virgin olive oil

Combine all ingredients except coconut and olive oils and mix well.

In a small bowl combine the coconut oil and olive oil, stirring well.

While whisking, slowly drizzle in the oil.

Nutritional breakdown per serving: 62 calories (96.0% from fat); 7 g fat; trace protein; 1 g carbohydrate; trace dietary fiber; 0 mg cholesterol; 78 mg sodium.

Curried Chicken Grape Salad

A delicious salad for lunch or dinner.

SERVES 4

½ cup Virgin Coconut Oil Mayonnaise (page 208) or mayonnaise
of choice
1 teaspoon fresh lemon juice
2 tablespoons curry powder
2 cups cooked chicken, chopped
¼ cup diced celery
½ cup Thompson seedless grapes, halved
¼ cup almond slivers
1 head Romaine lettuce

Blend mayonnaise, lemon juice, and curry powder.

Add the remaining ingredients (except lettuce) to a medium to
large salad bowl and toss with the mayonnaise mixture.

Chill at least 1 hour before serving.

Serve on a bed of whole leaves of Romaine lettuce.

Note: Walnuts may be substituted for almonds, and raisins (soaked
in hot water and drained) for grapes.

Nutritional breakdown per serving: 401 calories (61.1% from fat); 28 g fat; 28 g
protein; 12 g carbohydrate; 6 g dietary fiber; 111 mg cholesterol; 191 mg sodium.

SOUPS

Southwestern Black Bean Soup

This is a favorite in the Calbom household. Beans are a great source of fiber.

SERVES 4 TO 6

2 tablespoons virgin coconut oil
1 large onion, chopped
3 garlic cloves, minced
6 cups water
2 cups black beans, soaked overnight and drained, or
   3 (15-ounce) cans black beans, drained
1 cup fresh corn kernels, cut off the cob, or frozen corn
1 (4½-ounce) can diced green chilies or 2 tablespoons diced fresh
   mild green chili
¼ cup chopped cilantro
2 tablespoons tomato paste
1 teaspoon ground cumin
1 teaspoon dried oregano
½ teaspoon chili powder
Pinch freshly ground black pepper
1 teaspoon sea salt or Celtic salt

Garnish Options

Chopped cilantro
Minced onion
Plain yogurt or sour cream

In a large soup pot or Dutch oven, melt the coconut oil. Add the onion and garlic and sauté until tender. Add the water and the beans and bring to a boil. Reduce heat, cover, and simmer for 1½ hours or until the beans are tender. (If using canned beans, simmer for 30 minutes.)

Stir in the corn, chilies, cilantro, tomato paste, cumin, oregano, chili powder, and black pepper, and simmer, uncovered, for 30 minutes, or until the soup is somewhat thickened. The longer it simmers, the thicker the soup will be. Pour half or all the soup in a blender and puree, depending on taste. This will thicken the soup quickly and give it a nice, creamy consistency. Or, hold the corn until the soup is pureed, and then add. Add the salt at the very end and stir.

Pour the soup into bowls and top with your favorite garnishes.

Nutritional breakdown per serving: 270 calories (2% from fat); 5 g fat; 15 g protein; 51 g carbohydrate; 11 g dietary fiber; 0 mg cholesterol; 87 mg sodium.

Cream of 4-Mushroom Soup

Absolutely delicious!

SERVES 4

¼ to ½ pound button mushrooms
¼ pound oyster mushrooms (1 ounce dried, finely chopped)*
¼ pound shiitake mushrooms (1 ounce dried, finely chopped)
¼ pound porcini mushrooms (1 ounce dried, finely chopped)
2 whole shallots, minced
2 tablespoons virgin coconut oil
2 tablespoons unsalted butter
2 cups coconut milk; may use half coconut milk and half regular milk
4 egg yolks
1 cup heavy cream
½ cup sherry
Sea salt or Celtic salt, to taste
Black pepper, to taste

Clean fresh mushrooms, separating caps and stems. Set stems aside with reconstituted mushrooms. (If using dried mushrooms, reconstitute in hot water for about 20 to 30 minutes. Squeeze out excess water before slicing or chopping. Reconstituted mushrooms are better chopped finely.) If desired, slice half the fresh caps into ⅛-inch slices and set aside, add the remaining caps to the stems. Otherwise, combine caps and stems. Chop stems and remaining fresh caps very finely, set aside.

Peel and mince the shallots and set aside.

If using sliced mushroom caps, melt 1 tablespoon of the virgin coconut oil and 1 tablespoon of the unsalted butter in a stainless steel skillet over medium-high heat. When butter quits foaming, add sliced mushroom caps and sauté until they just turn color, about 5 minutes, remove from skillet and set aside. Add remaining virgin coconut oil and unsalted butter to skillet and when foaming stops, add chopped stems and caps and minced shallots and sauté until tender, about 10 minutes.

If not using sliced mushroom caps, melt the virgin coconut oil and unsalted butter in a stainless steel skillet. When foaming stops, add chopped stems and caps and minced shallots and sauté until tender, about 10 minutes.

Combine mushrooms and shallots with milk in a medium saucepan over medium-low heat; season with salt and pepper to taste. Simmer 20 to 25 minutes.

While mushrooms and coconut milk are simmering, whisk egg yolks until light and lemon colored. Whisk cream into eggs.

Whisk ½ cup of hot soup mixture into egg-cream mixture, two tablespoons at a time.

Then blend egg mixture into the rest of the soup, pouring in a slow, steady stream, and beating constantly.

Add sherry and reserved sliced mushroom caps, if used, and heat through, but do not allow to boil. Add salt and pepper.

*About 3 ounces of dried mushrooms is equivalent to 1 pound of fresh mushrooms. Use any combination of fresh or reconstituted dried mushrooms equivalent to 1 to 1¼ pounds of fresh mushrooms.

Nutritional breakdown per serving: 743 calories (82.6% from fat); 69 g fat; 10 g protein; 23 g carbohydrate; 5 g dietary fiber; 310 mg cholesterol; 62 mg sodium.

Tomato Basil Soup

A great soup that is easy to make.

SERVES 8

2 medium onions, diced
2 garlic cloves, chopped
1 tablespoon virgin coconut oil
5 small potatoes, peeled and diced
2 celery stalks, diced
¼ cup chopped parsley
2 tablespoons fresh basil leaves, chopped
1½ cups chicken broth
1 (28-ounce) can stewed tomatoes
2½ cups milk
Salt and pepper, to taste

Brown onions and garlic in oil for 3 to 4 minutes.

Mix in potato and celery dices, chopped parsley and basil.

Pour in chicken broth and tomatoes; simmer for 20 to 25 minutes, until vegetables are tender.

Pour in milk; reheat without boiling.

Salt and pepper, to taste. Puree into a blender.

Nutritional breakdown per serving: 160 calories (25.3% from fat); 5 g fat; 6 g protein; 25 g carbohydrate; 3 g dietary fiber; 14 mg cholesterol; 219 mg sodium.

VEGETABLE SIDE DISHES

Carrot-Pineapple Slaw

A tasty luncheon salad with a pineapple twist.

SERVES 8

4 cups shredded carrots
2 cups shredded cabbage
1 (16-ounce) can crushed pineapple in unsweetened juice,
  drained (reserve juice)
½ cup chopped walnuts
½ cup Virgin Coconut Oil Mayonnaise (page 208)
2 tablespoons low-carb healthy sweetener
2 tablespoons apple cider vinegar
½ teaspoon freshly ground black pepper

In large bowl, toss together carrots, cabbage, pineapple, and walnuts.

In small bowl, stir together remaining ingredients, including the reserved pineapple juice.

Pour dressing over slaw; toss gently. Cover and refrigerate 2 to 24 hours.

Nutritional breakdown per serving: 200 calories (61.7% from fat); 14 g fat; 3 g protein; 17 g carbohydrate; 3 g dietary fiber; 26 mg cholesterol; 80 mg sodium.

Butternut Squash, Sage, and Blue Cheese Gratin

A fabulous side dish that goes especially well with baked chicken.

SERVES 6

1 tablespoon virgin coconut oil
1¾ pounds butternut squash, 1 whole squash
1 tablespoon extra-virgin olive oil
1 tablespoon chopped fresh sage
¼ teaspoon sea salt or Celtic salt
¼ teaspoon freshly ground pepper
3 ounces crumbled blue cheese
1 ounce Gruyère cheese, shredded

Heat oven to 375 degrees F. Melt coconut oil in baking dish.

Cut squash in half lengthwise; remove seeds and peel. Slice each half crosswise into ½-inch-thick slices. Place squash in single layer at 45-degree angle in baking dish. (The squash will be tightly packed.)

Drizzle squash with olive oil. Sprinkle with sage, salt, and pepper. Cover with foil.

Bake 40 minutes or until squash is tender.

Remove from oven; remove foil.

Sprinkle with blue cheese and Gruyère cheese.

Return to oven; bake an additional 1 minute or until cheese is melted.

Nutritional breakdown per serving (excluding unknown items): 140 calories (48.5% from fat); 8 g fat; 6 g protein; 13 g carbohydrate; 2 g dietary fiber; 16 mg cholesterol; 296 mg sodium.

Caramelized Onion and Squash Gratin

SERVES 8

2 cups yellow onions, thinly sliced
2 tablespoons virgin coconut oil
6 cups acorn squash, peeled and coarsely grated
2 tablespoons whole wheat flour
2 tablespoons unsalted butter
2 teaspoons sea salt or Celtic salt, to taste
½ tablespoon white pepper, to taste
1½ cups Gruyère cheese, grated
1 cup half and half
½ cup whole wheat bread crumbs
⅓ cup grated Parmesan cheese
2 tablespoons chopped fresh parsley
2 tablespoons extra-virgin olive oil

Preheat oven to 375 degrees F.

Sauté the onions in the virgin coconut oil for 20 to 30 minutes or until golden, stirring often.

Spread 2 cups of the acorn squash in a baking dish. Layer with half the onions, flour, butter, salt, pepper, and Gruyère. Repeat.

Top with remaining squash. Pour half and half over the top. Combine the bread crumbs, Parmesan cheese, parsley, and olive oil. Sprinkle evenly over the top.

Bake for 35 to 40 minutes or until squash is tender and top is browned.

Nutritional breakdown per serving: 330 calories (56.3% from fat); 21 g fat; 11 g protein; 26 g carbohydrate; 4 g dietary fiber; 44 mg cholesterol; 739 mg sodium.

Roasted Squash with Poblano Pepper and Jack Cheese Quesadillas with Chipotle Lime Sour Cream

Make this dish, and you'll think you're dining in a fine restaurant.

SERVES 8

1 large butternut squash or 2 medium, peeled and cut into 1-inch chunks
1 large onion, unpeeled, cut into eighths
2 medium poblano peppers, seeded and halved
1 tablespoon vegetable oil
Sea salt or Celtic salt, to taste
Freshly ground black pepper
3 cloves garlic, minced
8 (8-inch) whole wheat flour tortillas
1 cup Monterey Jack Cheese, coarsely grated

Preheat oven to 400 degrees F.

In a shallow baking pan arrange squash, onion, and pepper in one layer and drizzle with oil, tossing to coat. Roast mixture in middle of oven for 20 to 30 minutes or until everything is tender. Do not let the bottom of the squash brown. Season with salt and pepper and add minced garlic.

In a food processor puree squash, onion, and pepper until smooth.

Spread about one-fourth squash puree on each of 4 tortillas and sprinkle each with about one-fourth of the cheese. Top each quesadilla with a plain tortilla, pressing gently together. Brush tops with oil.

Heat a griddle or nonstick skillet over moderately high heat until hot and cook quesadillas, one at a time until golden, about 3 minutes on each side.

Keep warm in a low oven while finishing with the rest of the quesadillas.

Transfer to a cutting board and cut into wedges.

Serve with Chipotle Lime Sour Cream Dip.

Quesadillas nutritional breakdown per serving: 410 calories (24% from fat); 11 g fat; 12 g protein; 68 g carbohydrate; 6 g dietary fiber; 13 mg cholesterol; 430 mg sodium.

Chipotle Lime Sour Cream Dip

Makes about 1 cup

1 chipotle chile canned in adobo, minced
2 teaspoons fresh lime juice
1 cup sour cream

In a small bowl stir chili and lime juice into sour cream until combined well. Make up to 2 days ahead, cover, and chill.

Dip nutritional breakdown per serving: 62 calories (85% from fat); 6 g fat; 1 g protein; 1 g carbohydrate; 0 g dietary fiber; 13 mg cholesterol; 27 mg sodium.

Wild Rice and Butternut Squash Pilaf

A delicious pilaf that could be the main dish.

Serves 6

¾ cup brown rice
¼ cup wild rice
2 tablespoons virgin coconut oil
2 medium onions, peeled and finely chopped
3 garlic cloves, minced
½ cup green or red bell pepper, chopped
⅓ pound button mushrooms, sliced
2½ cups chicken broth
1½ cups diced butternut squash
1 teaspoon dried thyme
½ teaspoon dried rosemary

1 tablespoon soy sauce
2 tablespoons dry sherry
¼ cup sliced almonds, lightly toasted
1 tablespoon chopped fresh parsley, for garnish

In a large, ungreased skillet, toast the rice over medium heat, stirring frequently, for 3 to 5 minutes. Do *not* let the rice burn. Set aside.

In a Dutch oven or large saucepan, heat the oil over medium heat, add the onions, garlic, pepper, and mushrooms; sauté the vegetables until softened, approximately 8 to 10 minutes.

Add the toasted rice to the vegetable mixture along with the broth, squash, thyme, rosemary, soy sauce, and sherry.

Bring the mixture to a boil, reduce the heat, cover the pan, and simmer for 40 to 60 minutes or until the liquid is absorbed and the rice is tender.

Toss the rice with the toasted almonds before serving the pilaf. Garnish with the fresh parsley.

Nutritional breakdown per serving: 211 calories (19.9% from fat); 5 g fat; 8 g protein; 35 g carbohydrate; 3 g dietary fiber; 0 mg cholesterol; 496 mg sodium.

Thai Green Vegetable Curry

Another authentic Thai dish that will make your mouth water.

SERVES 3 TO 4

Homemade Coconut Milk (page 206) or 1 (13.5-ounce) can
 coconut milk
½ tablespoon green curry paste, or to taste
1 tablespoon virgin coconut oil
4 kaffir lime leaves, optional
1 cup chopped onion
2 cups broccoli, stems peeled and sliced and tops separated into
 flowerets

2 medium carrots, thinly sliced
1½ cups cauliflower flowerets
½ bell pepper, sliced
¼ cup fresh basil leaves
2 cups cooked brown jasmine rice
Fresh cilantro leaves, for garnish

Pour the coconut milk into a Dutch oven. Add the curry paste, to taste, and the coconut oil. Simmer, covered, for about 5 minutes.

Add the kaffir lime leaves, if using, then add the onion and the broccoli stems. Simmer for about 2 minutes more.

Add the remaining ingredients, except for the basil, rice, and cilantro. Simmer covered for 10 to 15 minutes, or until the vegetables are just tender.

Stir in the basil leaves, and serve immediately over brown jasmine rice. Garnish with cilantro.

Nutritional breakdown per serving (based on 4 servings): 595 calories (36% from fat); 24 g fat; 12 g protein; 87 g carbohydrate; 0 mg cholesterol; 53 mg sodium.

MEAT, FISH, AND CHICKEN ENTRÉES

Garlic-Parmesan Halibut

This halibut is so delicious it's hard to believe that it's a healthy, low-carb entrée.

SERVES 4 TO 6

1 to 1½ pounds halibut, cut into 4 pieces
¼ cup fresh lemon juice
Black pepper, to taste
Sea salt or Celtic salt, to taste

Topping

2 tablespoons Virgin Coconut Oil Mayonnaise (page 208), or mayonnaise of choice
2 tablespoons finely grated Parmesan cheese
2 tablespoons fresh lemon juice
2 tablespoons finely chopped green onions
2 garlic cloves, pressed or finely chopped
1 teaspoon Dijon mustard
¼ teaspoon hot sauce or pinch of cayenne pepper
Sea salt or Celtic salt, to taste

Preheat oven to 450 degrees F.

On each side of the fish steak, make 3 diagonal cuts 2 inches long and ½ inch deep. Place the halibut in a large, shallow dish and pour the lemon juice over it; marinate for 30 minutes at room temperature.

Place the fish on a broiling pan and sprinkle with lemon juice from the marinade along with black pepper. Bake the fish for 15 minutes, or until it is opaque in the middle.

While the halibut is baking, combine the mayonnaise, Parmesan cheese, lemon juice, green onions, garlic, mustard, and hot sauce or cayenne in a small bowl and mix well.

Remove halibut from the oven and then turn the oven to broil.

Sprinkle salt, as desired, over the fish and then spread some of the topping over each filet. Broil the fish for about 1 minute, or until the topping is golden brown.

Nutritional breakdown per serving (based on 6 servings): 167 calories (30% from fat); 3 g fat; 24 g protein; 2 g carbohydrate; 58 mg cholesterol; 132 mg sodium.

Resources

WEBSITES FOR CHERIE CALBOM, M.S.

www.gococonuts.com—Information on the authors, the Coconut Diet, and virgin coconut oil

Other websites of Cherie Calbom, M.S.—www.juicinginfo.net, www.cleansing info.com, and www.ultimatesmoothie.com, www.cancercleanse.net, and www.wrinklecleanse.net

Tel: 866-8GETWEL/866-843-8935

NATURAL HEALTH WEBSITE

www.mercola.com—Natural health website by Dr. Joseph Mercola

BOOKS

Note: all these books can be ordered at www.gococonuts.com

The Cholesterol Myths (New Trends Publishing) by Uffe Ravnskov, M.D., Ph.D.

The Juice Lady's Guide to Juicing for Health (Avery) by Cherie Calbom

Know Your Fats: The Complete Primer for Understanding the Nutrition of Fats, Oils, and Cholesterol (Bethesda Press) by Mary G. Enig, Ph.D.

Patient Heal Thyself (Freedom Press) by Jordan Rubin

The Ultimate Smoothie Book (Warner Books) by Cherie Calbom

The Whole Soy Story (New Trends Publishing) by Kaayla T. Daniel

The Wrinkle Cleanse (Avery) by Cherie Calbom

The Complete Cancer Cleanse (Thomas Nelson) by Cherie Calbom, John Calbom, and Michael Mahaffey

SOURCES OF COCONUT PRODUCTS

Coconut Oil

Expeller Pressed Coconut Oil
www.gococonuts.com
Tel: 866-8GETWEL

Organic Virgin Coconut Oil
www.gococonuts.com
Tel: 866-8GETWEL

Coconut Cream and Milk

Coconut Cream Concentrate
www.gococonuts.com
Tel: 866-8GETWEL

SOURCES OF OTHER FOOD PRODUCTS

Cod Liver Oil

Carlson's Cod Liver Oil
Health food stores

Sugar

Pure Birch Sugar—The Ultimate Sweetener, 800-843-6325

EXERCISES

- *Walk Away the Pounds* by Leslie Sansone; book and video (NY: Warner, 2005)
- Lymphasizer (Swing Machine) www.juicinginfo.com or 866-8GETWEL

SOURCES OF CLEANSE PRODUCTS

Colon Cleans

Advanced Naturals: Fiber Max, Colon Cleanse I and II
Arise & Shine Products: Psyllium, Bentonite, Herbal Nutrition, and Chomper
Dr. Schultz's Intestinal Formula #1 and #2

Candida albicans Cleanse Products

Candida Cleanse—Silver Creek Labs, 800-493-1146

Kidney Cleanse Herbs

Kidney Life—Arise & Shine, 866-8GETWEL

Liver Cleanse Herbs

Liver Life I and II, 866-8GETWEL
Liver Cleanse (Thorne), 866-8GETWEL

Parasite Cleanse Products

Dr. Schultz's Liver Cleanse

SOURCES OF SUPPLEMENTS AND RELATED PRODUCTS

Juice Concentrates

Black Cherry Juice Concentrate—Dynamic Health (can be found at many health food stores)

Cranberry Juice Concentrate—Dynamic Health (can be found at many health food stores)

Elderberry Juice Concentrate—Natural Sources (can be found at many health food stores)

Lipotropic Formula (helpful for liver and gallbladder cleansing)

Lipo-Gen—Metagenics, 866-8GETWEL

Minerals

Bio Available Liquid Minerals—Eniva Essentials, 866-8GETWEL

Probiotics

Ultra Flora Plus DF Capsules—Metagenics, 866-8GETWEL

Rice Protein

Ultra Inflam X, 866-8GETWEL

Thyroid and Adrenal Support

Adrenal Support: Androgen
Metagenics
Tel: 866-8GETWEL

Liquid Iodine
Biotics Research
Tel: 866-8GETWEL

Thyroid Support: Thyrosol
Metagenics
Tel: 866-8GETWEL

HEALTH CENTERS

The following centers offer a raw foods/juice detoxification program. They offer nutritional classes and some offer other health classes that address the emotional, mental, and spiritual aspects of health and renewal. In addition, most of the centers offer massage and colonics. It is best to contact the various centers to find out which one best fits your needs.

Cedar Springs Renewal Center
Michael Mahaffey and Nan Monk, Directors
31459 Barben Road
Sedro Woolley, WA 98284
Tel: 360-826-3599
Fax: 360-422-1524
Website: www.cedarsprings.org

HealthQuarters Ministries
David Frahm, N.D., Director
3620 W. Colorado Avenue
Colorado Springs, CO 80904
Tel: 719-593-8694
Fax: 719-531-7884
E-mail: healthqu@healthquarters.org
Website: healthquarters.org

Hippocrates Institute
Brian and Anna Maria Clement, Directors
1443 Palmdale Court
West Palm Beach, FL 33411
Tel: 800-842-2125
Fax: 561-471-9464
E-mail: hippocrates@worldnet.att.net
Website: www.hippocratesinstitute.org

Optimum Health Institute of Austin
265 Cedar Drive
Cedar Creek, TX 78612
Tel: 512-303-4817
Fax: 512-303-1239
E-mail: austin@optimumhealth.org
Website: www.optimumhealth.org

Optimum Health Institute of San Diego
6970 Central Avenue
Lemon Grove, CA 91945-2198
Tel: 800-993-4325
Fax: 619-589-4098
E-mail: optimum@optimumhealth.org
Website: www.optimumhealth.org

Sanoviv Medical Institute
Dr. Myron Wentz, Director
Playa de Rosarito, Km 39
Baja, California, Mexico
Tel: 800-726-6848
Fax: 801-954-7477
Website: www.sanoviv.com

We Care
Susana and Susan Lombardi, Directors
18000 Long Canyon Road
Desert Hot Springs, CA 92241
Tel: 800-888-2523
Fax: 760-251-5399
E-mail: info@wecarespa.com
Website: www.wecarespa.com

HEALTHY COOKING CLASSES

Edith Carter, the Healthy Gourmet
Edith has personally taught over 1,000 students how to make healthy food taste delicious. She is frequently in demand as a speaker at health industry events and has written several cookbooks. She works closely with leading health industry professionals to spread the message that eating well can be tasty and nutritious.
The Healthy Company
Website: www.thehealthygourmet.com

Vicki Chelf, Cooking Classes and Gourmet Club

Vicki teaches classes on healthy cooking and has written several books, including *Cooking on the Right Side of the Brain.*

E-mail: vrchelf@hotmail.com

PERSONAL CHEF

Chef Pierre

Pete V. McCracken

Tel: 559-784-2341

E-mail: PersonalChef@cwdi.org

Notes

CHAPTER 1

1. Y. Y. Yeh and P. Zee, "Relation of ketosis in metabolic changes induced by acute medium-chain triglyceride feeding in rats." *J Nutr.* 106 (1976): 58–67.

2. B. I. Bloom, L. L. Chaikoff, and W. O. Reinhardt, "Intestinal Lymph as Pathway for Transport of Absorbed Fatty Acids of Different Lengths," *Am. J. Physiology* 166 (1951): 451–455; J. R. Senior, ed., *Medium Chain Triglycerides* (Philadelphia: University of Pennsylvania Press, 1968), pp. 3–6; A. C. Bach and U. K. Babyan, "Medium Chain Triglycerides: An update," *Am. J. Clin. Nutr.* 36 (1982): 950–962.

3. J. H. Wiley and G. A. Leveille, "Metabolic consequences of dietary medium-chain triglycerides in the rat." *J Nutr* 103 (1973): 829–835. A. Geliebter, N. Torbay, E. F. Bracco, et al., "Overfeeding with medium-chain triglyceride diet results in diminished deposition of fat." *Am. J. Clin. Nutr.* 37 (1983): 1–4. S. A. Hashim, "Dietary fats and adipose tissue fatty acid composition." *Prev Med* 12 (1983): 854–867.

4. N. Baba, E. F. Bracco, S. A. Hashim, "Enhanced thermogenesis and diminished deposition of fat in response to overfeeding with diet containing medium-chain triglyceride. *Am. J. Clin. Nutr.* 35 (1982): 678–682. T. B. Seaton, S. L. Welle, M. K. Warenko, et al., "Thermic effects of medium-chain and long-chain triglycerides in man. *Am. J. Clin. Nutr.* 44 (1986): 630–634. J. O. Hill, J. C. Peters, D. Yang, et al., "Thermogenesis in humans during overfeeding with medium-chain triglycerides." *Metabolism* 38 (1989): 641–648.

5. I. A. Prior, F. Davidson, C. E. Salmond, and Z. Czochanska, "Cholesterol, Coconuts, and Diet on Polynesian Atolls: A Natural Experiment: The Pukapuka and Tokelau Island Studies," *Am. J. Clin. Nutr.* 34(8) (1981): 1552–1561; Bruce Fife, N.D., *The Healing Miracles of Coconut Oil* (Colorado Springs, CO: HealthWise, 2001), pp. 20–23.

6. J. J. Kabara, "Health Oils from the Tree of Life" (Nutritional and Health Aspects of Coconut Oil), *Indian Coconut Journal* 31(8) (2000): 2–8.

7. Mary G. Enig, Ph.D., "Health and Nutritional Benefits from Coconut Oil: An Important Functional Food for the 21st Century," Presented at the AVOC Lauric Oils Symposium, Ho Chi Minh City, Vietnam, April 25, 1996.

8. "In Vitro Killing of *Candida albicans* by Fatty Acids and Monoglycerides," *Antimicrobial Agents Chemother* 45(11) (November 2001): 3209–3212.

9. Weston Price, *Nutrition and Physical Degeneration* (Keats Publishing, 1998).

10. S. Sircar and U. Kansra, Department of Medicine, Safdarjang Hospital, New Delhi. "Choice of Cooking Oils—Myths and Realities," *J. Indian Med. Assoc.* 96(10) (October 1998): 304–307.

11. P. K. Thampan, *Facts and Fallacies About Coconut Oil,* Asian and Pacific Coconut Community, Jakarta, 1994.

12. Dr. P. Rethinam and Muhartoyo, "The Plain Truth About Coconut Oil," *Jakarta Post,* June 18, 2003/www.apccsec.org/truth.html.

13. H. Kaunitz, "Medium Chain Triglycerides (MCT) in Aging and Arteriosclerosis," *J. Environ. Pathol. Toxicol. Oncol.* 6(3–4) (March–April 1986): 115–121.

14. Dr. Mary Enig has written two articles—"The Oiling of America" and "Coconut: In Support of Good Health in the 21st Century"—that provide an in-depth analysis of saturated fat research and the negative campaigns that have been waged against coconut oil. This history of the edible oil industry in the United States has been well documented by Doctor Enig, and can be reviewed at www.coconutoil.com or the Weston A. Price Foundation website at www.westonaprice.org. See also Bruce Fife, N.D., *The Healing Miracles of Coconut Oil* (Colorado Springs, CO: Piccadilly Books, 2003), pp. 26–32.

15. Bruce Fife, p. 27.

16. Mary G. Enig, "Coconut: In Support of Good Health in the 21st Century," presented at the Asian Pacific Coconut Community's 36th Session, 1999.

17. Mary G. Enig, "Coconut: In Support of Good Health in the 21st Century."

18. Bruce Fife, p. 28.

CHAPTER 2

1. Ron Rosedale, M.D., "Insulin and Its Metabolic Effects," p. 6. Available at www.mercola.com.

2. Ron Rosedale, p. 5.

3. A conversation that Dr. Robert C. Atkins had with Brenda Watson, author of *Renew Life* and *Gut Solutions.* As told to Cherie Calbom, February 2004.

4. Nikki and David Goldbeck, *The Goldbecks' Guide to Good Food* (New York: New American Library, 1987), pp. 420–433.

5. L. J. Forristal, "The Murky World of High Fructose Corn Syrup," *Wise Traditions* 2(3) (2001): 60–61.
6. Miryam Ehrlich Williamson, *Blood Sugar Blues* (New York: Walker & Company, 2001), p. 136.
7. H. J. Roberts, M.D., "Does Aspartame Cause Human Brain Cancer?" *J. Advance. of Med.* 4(4) (Winter 1991): 231–241.
8. "Aspartame and Dieting," *Nutrition Week* 27(23) (June 13, 1997): 7j *Int. J. Obes.* 21(1) (January, 1997): 37–42.
9. Cheryl R. Hart, M.D., and Mary Kay Grossman, R.D., *The Insulin-Resistance Diet* (Chicago: Contemporary Books, 2001), pp. 73–74.
10. Cheryl R. Hart and Mary Kay Grossman, pp. 73–75.
11. E. N. Anderson Jr. and M. L. Anderson, *Modern China South,* (1977), pp. 317–382.
12. Jennie Brond-Miller, Susana Holt, Kay Foster-Powell, and Johanna Burani, *The New Glucose Revolution: Complete Guide to Glycemic Index Values* (Berkeley, CA: Pub Group West, 2003).
13. Ron Rosedale, p. 6.
14. Ron Rosedale, p. 5.
15. Ron Rosedale, p. 2.
16. Cheryl R. Hart and Mary Kay Grossman, p. 173.
17. Nicholas Perricone, M.D., *The Perricone Prescription* (New York: Harper Resource, 2002), pp. 12, 173.
18. Nicholas Perricone, pp. 12, 173.
19. T. A. Mori, et al., "Dietary Fish as a Major Component of a Weight-Loss Diet: Effect on Serum Lipids, Glucose, and Insulin Metabolism in Overweight Hypertensive Subjects," *Am. J. Clin. Nutr.* 70 (1999): 817–825.
20. Cheryl R. Hart and Mary Kay Grossman, p. 19.

CHAPTER 3

1. National Health and Nutrition Examination Survey 1999–2000.
2. Centers for Disease Control and Prevention/www.cdc.gov
3. Gary Taubes, "What If It's All Been a Big Fat Lie?" *New York Times* magazine, July 7, 2002.
4. Rex Russell, M.D., *What the Bible Says About Healthy Living* (Ventura, CA: Regal Books, 1996), p. 125.
5. B. A. Watkins, et al., "Importance of Vitamin E in Bone Formation and in Chrondrocyte Function," Purdue University, Lafayette, IN, AOCS Proceedings, 1996; B. A. Watkins and M. F. Seifert, "Food Lipids and Bone Health," in *Food Lipids and Health,* R. E. McDonald and D. B. Min, eds. (New York, Marcel Dekker, 1996), p. 101.

6. G. H. Dahlen, et al., *J. Intern. Med.* 244(5) (November 1998): 417–424; P. Khosla and K. C. Hayes, *J. Am. Coll. Nutr.* 15 (1996): 325–339; B. A. Clevidence, et al., *Arterioscler. Thromb. Vasc. Biol.* 17 (1997): 1657–1661.

7. A. A. Nanji, et al., *Gastroenterology* 109(2) (August 1995): 547–554; Y. S. Cha and D. S. Sachan, *J. Am. Coll. Nutr.* 13(4) (August 1994): 338–343; H. L. Hargrove, et al., *FASEB Journal,* Meeting Abstracts 204.1 (March 1999): A222.

8. J. J. Kabara, *The Pharamacological Effects of Lipids* (Champaign, IL: The American Oil Chemists Society, 1978), pp. 1–14; L. A. Cohen, et al., *J. Natl. Cancer Inst.* 77 (1986): 43.

9. M. L. Garg, et al., *FASEB Journal* 2(4) (1988): A852; R. M. Oliart Ros, et al. "Meeting Abstracts," AOCS Proceedings, May 1998, p. 7, Chicago, IL.

10. L. D. Lawson and F. Kummerow, *Lipids* 14 (1979): 501–503; M. L. Garg, *Lipids* 24(4) (April 1989): 334–339.

11. *Ugeskr Laeger,* 166(1–2) (January 5, 2004): 29–32.

12. FDA website: http://fda.gov.

13. N. Baba, E. F. Bracco, and S. A. Hashim, "Enhanced Thermogenesis and Diminished Deposition of Fat in Response to Overfeeding with Diet Containing Medium Chain Triglycerides." *Am. J. Clin. Nutr.* 35(4) (April 1982): 678–682.

14. *Raymond Peat Newsletter,* "Unsaturated Vegetable Oils Toxic" (1996 edition): p. 2.

15. J. O. Hill, J. C. Peters, D. Yang, T. Sharp, M. Kaler, N. N. Abumrad, and H. L. Greene, "Thermogenesis in Humans During Overfeeding with Medium-Chain Triglycerides," *Metabolism* 38(7) (July 1989): 641–648.

16. M. P. St-Onge, R. Ross, W. D. Parsons, and P. J. Jones, "Medium-Chain Triglycerides Increase Energy Expenditure and Decrease Adiposity in Overweight Men," *Obes. Res.* 11(3) (March 2003): 395–402.

17. Mary G. Enig, Ph.D., *Know Your Fats* (Silver Springs, MD: Bethesda Press, 2000), p. 46.

18. Mary G. Enig, p. 107.

19. G. Crozier, B. Bois-Joyeux, M. Chanex, et al., "Overfeeding with Medium-Chain Triglycerides in the Rat," *Metabolism* 36 (1987): 807–814.

20. T. B. Seaton, S. L. Welles, M. K. Warenko, et al., "Thermic Effects of Medium-Chain and Long-Chain Triglycerides in Man." *Am. J. Clin. Nutr.* 44 (1986): 630–634.

21. S. A. Hashim, "Dietary Fats and Adipose Tissue Fatty Acid Composition," *Prev. Med.* 12 (1983): 854–867.

22. "Heart Guidelines Urge Test for Inflammation," *USA Today,* January 28, 2003.

23. Mary Enig, Ph.D., "Health and Nutritional Benefits from Coconut Oil: An

Important Functional Food in the 21st Century," Presented at the AVOC Lauric Oils Symposium, Ho Chi Minh City, Vietnam, April 25, 1996.

24. Mary Enig.

25. J. H. Wiley and G. A. Leveille, "Metabolic Consequences of Dietary Medium Chain Triglycerides in the Rat." *J. Nutr.* 103 (1973): 829–835.

26. C. V. Felton, D. Crook, M. J. Davies, and M. F. Oliver, Wynn Institute for Metabolic Research, London, UK. "Dietary Polyunsaturated Fatty Acids and Composition of Human Aortic Plaques," *Lancet* 29:344(8931) (October 1994): 1195–1196.

27. J. W. Eikelboom, et al., "Homocyst(e)ine and Cardiovascular Disease: A Critical Review of the Epidemiological Evidence," *Ann. Intern. Med.* 131(5) (September 7, 1999): 363–375.

28. S. Morris, et al., "Hyperhomocysteinemia and Hypercholesterolemia Associated with Hypothyroidism in the Third U.S. National Health and Nutrition Examination Survey," *Atherosclerosis* 155 (2001): 195–200.

CHAPTER 4

1. Gay J. Canaris, M.D., M.S.P.H., Neil R. Manowitz, Ph.D., Gilbert Mayor, M.D., and E. Chester Ridgway, M.D. "The Colorado Thyroid Disease Prevalence Study," *Arch. Intern. Med.* 160 (2000): 526–534.

2. Kenneth Blanchard, M.D., *What Your Doctor May Not Tell You About Hypothyroidism* (New York: Warner, 2004).

3. Ridha Arem, *The Thyroid Solution: A Mind-Body Program for Beating Depression and Regaining Your Emotional and Physical Health* (New York: Ballantine Books, 1999).

4. L. A. G. Ries, M. A. Smith, J. G. Gurney, M. Linet, T. Tamra, J. L. Young, and G. R. Bunin, eds., *Cancer Incidence and Survival Among Children and Adolescents: United States SEER Program 1975–1995,* National Cancer Institute, SEER Program (Bethesda, MD: NIH Pub. No. 99-4649, 1999), Chapter: "Carcinomas and Other Malignant Epithelial Neoplasms," Leslie Bernstein and James G. Gurney.

5. L. A. G. Ries, M. A. Smith, J. G. Gurney, M. Linet, T. Tamra, J. L. Young, and G. R. Bunin, eds., *Cancer Incidence and Survival Among Children and Adolescents: United States SEER Program 1975–1995,* National Cancer Institute, SEER Program. (Bethesda, MD: NIH Pub. No. 99-4649, 1999).

6. *Raymond Peat Newsletter,* "Unsaturated Vegetable Oils Toxic" (1996), p. 4.

7. P. Fort, N. Moses, M. Fasano, T. Goldberg, and F. Lifshitz, "Breast and Soy— Formula Feeding in Early Infancy and the Prevalence of Autoimmune Thyroid Disease in Children," *J. Am. Col. Nutr.* (9) (1990): 164–167.

8. Daniel R. Doerge, Hebron C. Chang, "Inactivation of thyroid peroxidase by

soy isoflavones in vitro and in vivo." *J. Chromotography B* 777(1,2):25 (September 2002): 269–79.

9. M. T. See and J. Odle, "Effect of Dietary Fat Source, Level, and Feeding Interval on Pork Fatty Acid Composition." 1998–2000 Department Report, Department of Animal Science, ANS Report No. 248; North Carolina State University.

10. *Raymond Peat Newsletter,* "Unsaturated Vegetable Oils Toxic," p. 5.

11. David Frähm, *Health Quarters Monthly,* Vol. 58, August 2003.

12. *The Journal of Biochemistry* (79:409–11; 1928) in John Heinerman, *Heinerman's Encyclopedia of Healing Juices* (Englewood Cliffs, NJ: Prentice Hall, 1994), p. 49.

13. This article is adapted from Cherie Calbom, M.S. "Thyroid Health: A Key to Weight Loss," Issue 479 (November 8, 2003), available at www.mercola.com.

CHAPTER 5

1. As told to Cherie Calbom in a conversation with Brenda Watson, N.D., author of *Renew Life* and *Gut Solutions,* February 2004. This information was part of a conversation Brenda had with the late Dr. Robert C. Atkins.

2. William G. Crook, M.D., *The Yeast Connection* (Jackson, TN: Professional Books, 1983), p. 14.

3. O. Truss, *The Missing Diagnosis* (Birmingham, AL, P.O. Box 26508, 1983) in Michael Murray, N.D., and Joseph Pizzorno, N.D., *Encyclopedia of Natural Medicine* (Rocklin, CA: Prima Publishing, 1998), p. 300.

4. G. F. Kroker, "Chronic Candidiasis and Allergy," in *Food Allergy and Intolerance,* J. Brostoff and S. J. Challacombe, eds. (Philadelphia: W. B. Saunders, 1987), pp. 850–872; Michael Murray and Joseph Pizzorno, *Encyclopedia of Natural Medicine* pp. 300, 306.

5. Gudmundur Bergsson, Jóhann Arnfinnsson, Ólafur Steingrímsson, and Halldor Thormar, "In Vitro Killing of Candida albicans by Fatty Acids and Monoglycerides," *Antimicro. Agents and Chemother.* 45(11) (November 2001): pp. 3209–3212. Institute of Biology, University of Iceland, Department of Anatomy, University of Iceland Medical School, and Department of Microbiology, National University Hospital, Reykjavik, Iceland.

6. Michael Murray and Joseph Pizzorno, *Encyclopedia of Natural Medicine,* pp. 306–8; F. Abe, S. Nagata, and M. Hotchi, "Experimental Candidiasis in Liver Injury," *Mycopathologica* 100 (1987): 37–42.

7. Michael Murray and Joseph Pizzorno, p. 127.

8. Thampan, P. K., *Facts and Fallacies About Coconut Oil* (Asian and Pacific Coconut Community [1994]), p. 8.

9. G. K. Adler, et al., "Reduced Hypothalmic-Pituitary and Sympathoadrenal

Responses to Hypoglycemia in Women with Fibromyalgia Syndrome," *Am. J. Med.* 106 (May 1999): 534–543.

10. Cherie Calbom, John Calbom, and Michael Mahaffey, *The Complete Cancer Cleanse* (Nashville, TN: Thomas Nelson Publishers, 2003), pp. 66–68; adapted from John Calbom "The Choice Response: Changing Your Eating Habits," *Body, Mind and Spirit; Choices.* November 1992.

CHAPTER 6

1. Norine Dworkin, "Can't Lose Weight?" *Family Circle,* March 9, 2004, p. 112.
2. Julian Whitaker, *Health & Healing* 14(1) (January 2004).
3. IT Services, "Nutritional Quality: Organic vs. Conventional," *Clinical Pearls: The Experts Speak* (2001): 116.
4. V. Worthington, "Nutritional Quality of Organic Versus Conventional Fruits, Vegetables, and Grains," *Journal of Alternative and Complementary Medicine* 72(2) (2001): 161–173.
5. Michael Murray, N.D., and Joseph Pizzorno, N.D., *Encyclopedia of Natural Medicine* (Rocklin, CA: Prima Publishing, 1998), pp. 476–484.

CHAPTER 7

1. Shonagh Walker, *Cellulite: Not Just a Fancy Name for Fat* (Sydney, Australia: HarperCollins, 2001), pp. 42–43.
2. Shonagh Walker, pp. 42–43.
3. Shonagh Walker (from an interview about her book with Bronwen Gora, *Thigh Anxiety*).
4. Shonagh Walker (from an interview about her book with Bronwen Gora, *Thigh Anxiety*).
5. Brenda Watson and Leonard Smith, *Gut Solutions* (Clearwater, FL: Renew Life, 2003), p. 170.
6. David Frähm, *Health Quarters Monthly* 63 (January 2004): 2.

Acknowledgments

I wish to express my deep and lasting appreciation to all the people who have assisted me with this book, especially Brian and Marianita Shilhavy, who lent their expertise on coconut oil and the traditional coconut diet to me as I prepared this manuscript. All the testimonies in this book are from clients of Tropical Traditions virgin coconut oil, and were taken from the Internet Discussion Group of Tropical Traditions at www.coconutdiet.com. To Vicki Chelf, friend and coauthor of *Cooking for Life,* who created a number of scrumptious recipes for Phases III and IV, as always, you're the best! Special thanks also goes to Edith Carter, known as The Healthy Gourmet, who created many fabulous recipes found in Phase I. And, my special thanks also goes to Chef Pierre, Personal Chef Services, who created a number of delectable recipes for Phase I, III, and IV. A very special thanks goes to my literary agent, Pamela Harty, who walked the road of challenges with me every step of this project. You are one of God's gifts to me and I'm so glad I found you. To my editor, Diana Baroni, I am so grateful for your creative input and good-natured suggestions; you helped make this book extra special. And thanks as well to Leila Porteous for your help on edits and your cheerful responses. To John, my husband and coauthor—you're such great support and my very best friend. And most of all to God, who answered many prayers concerning this project, I offer my eternal gratitude.

—Cherie Calbom

To my lovely wife, Cherie, whose passion for helping people gain a better measure of health, I wish to offer my deepest gratitude. Once again, you've encouraged me to share my insights. Thank you for spurring me on. And to our chefs, the Shilhavys, our agent and editors—Cherie summed it up, and I add my gratitude and thanks.

—John Calbom

Index

1-Day Colon Cleanse, menu plan, 218, 219
1-Day Vegetable Juice Cleanse, 132–33
7-Day Gallbladder Flush, 229–32
7-Day Healthy Carbs, menu plan, 242–46
7-Day Kidney Flush, 233
7-Day Liver Cleanse, 76, 224–28
7-Day Weight Maintenance, menu plan, 276–80
21-Day Weight Loss Diet, ix, 16, 113–212
   Daily Food Log, 114, 152
   foods to avoid, 128–31
   foods to eat, 117–27
   juicing, 131–34
   menu plan, 136–51
   recipes, 153–212

Abdominal pain, gallstones and, 229
Acorn squash, recipes, 262–63, 291
Actos, 33
Adrenal glands, 92
Aerobic exercise, 37, 76–77, 116
Alcohol, 29, 75, 128, 223, 274
Allergies, 84, 217
Almond milk, recipes, 207, 268–69
American Heart Association, 54
American Soybean Association (ASA), 14
Animal protein, 113, 118, 122–23
   to avoid, 128, 274
   blood sugar and, 37
   CLA levels and, 50–51
   heart disease and, 56
Antibiotics, 9–10, 83

Antifungals, 87
Antioxidants, 86, 114, 133
Arem, Ridha, 61–62
Arthritis, 68
Artificial sweeteners, 27–29, 35–36
Aspartame, 28
Atkins, Robert C. (Atkins diet), 22, 82
Avocados, 125
   recipes, 134–35, 251–52, 282–83

Barnes, Broda, 56–57
Beans. See Legumes
Beets, 30
   recipes, 170–71, 226, 232
Beta carotene, 30, 73
Beverages, 118–19, 123–24
   to avoid, 128, 274
Bile, 90, 135, 223, 228, 229
Birch sugar, 23
Black bean soup, recipe, 285–86
Blackburn, George, 14
Black cherry juice, 220, 300
Blanchard, Kenneth, 61
Blood sugar (glucose), 29–34
   cravings and, 31–32
   glycemic index and, 29–31, 92
   sweeteners and, 24, 28
Blood vessels, cellulite and, 215
Body temperature, 60–61, 68
Books, recommended, 297
Breads. See Grains
Breakfast recipes, 153–62, 247–48, 281–83

Brown rice syrup, 24
Brown sugar, 26
Butter, 124, 125
Butternut squash, recipes, 290, 292–94

Caffeine. *See* Coffee
Calcium, 70
Cancer, thyroid, 62
Candida Questionnaire, 22, 87, 101–6
Candidiasis, 82–89
    correcting the problem, 84–87
    Herxheimer reaction, 87–88
    predisposing factors, 83
    resources, 299
    sugar cravings and, 22, 32
Capric acid, 84
Caprylic acid, 84
Carbohydrates (carbs), 17–40. *See also* Healthy
        carbs; Sweeteners
    complex, 20–21, 37
    simple, 18–20, 22, 29, 37, 41–43
    worst, 18–20, 29
Carrots, 232
    recipes, 167–68, 226, 258, 267, 289
Cellulite, 215–16, 223
Celtic salt, 72, 127
Center for Science in the Public Interest
        (CSPI), 14
Cheeses, 118, 119
    to avoid, 128–29, 237, 274
    recipes, 157, 266, 282–83, 290, 292–93
    reintroducing to diet, 236
Chicken, 118, 122–23, 274. *See also* Recipes
Cholesterol, 12–13, 53–56
Chromium, 32
Chronic candidiasis, 83
Chronic fatigue syndrome, 87, 92–94
CLA (conjugated linoleic acid), 50–51
Cleansing, x, 76, 213–34
    1-Day Vegetable Juice Cleanse, 132–33, 220
    chronic fatigue syndrome and, 93
    digestive disorders and, 90–91
    how it works, 213–14
    resources, 299–300
Coconut oil, overview, vii–ix, 3–16
Coconut products, resources, 298
Cod liver oil, 53, 73, 136, 299
Coffee
    to avoid, 128, 136, 274
    insulin sensitivity and, 36
    liver function and, 223
    thyroid function and, 75

Colon cleansing, 214, 216–22
    candida and, 87
    menu plan, 219
    recipes and products, 219–20, 299
Colonics, 221–22
Comfort foods, 95–96
Complex carbohydrates, 20–21, 37
Conjugated linoleic acid (CLA), 50–51
Constipation, 90, 217
Cooking classes, resources, 303
Cooking techniques, basic, 239–41
Corn, 48–49, 52
Corn oil, 47, 48, 54
Corn syrup, 27
Cortisone (cortisol), 31–32, 36, 116–17
Cranberry juice, 74, 234, 300
Cravings, 20, 31–32, 114–15
Crohn's disease, 90
Crook, William, 84, 87
Curries, recipes, 260–62, 265, 294–95

Daily Food Log, 114, 152
Dairy. *See* Cheeses; Milk and dairy
Date sugar, 25
Detoxification. *See* Cleansing
Dextrose, 27
Diabetes, 33, 34
Digestive disorders, 85, 89–91
Dinner recipes, 183–206, 259–63,
    295–96
Disaccharides, 18
Diverticular disease, 90
Drinking, 29, 75, 128, 223, 274
Dysbiosis, 90

Eating habits, 97–100
Eggplant, recipes, 192–93, 201–2
Eggs, 72, 119, 122. *See also* Recipes
Emotional eating, 94–100
Endorphins, 115–16
Enig, Mary, 13, 14, 53, 54–55
Epinephrine, 38
Epstein-Barr virus, 92, 94
Equal, 28
Essential fatty acids, 36, 37, 48–55, 122
Exercise, 37, 76–77, 115–16
    resources, 299

Fasting, 87
Fatigue, 87, 92–94

Fats, 38, 41–58
  to avoid, 57–58, 274–75
  cellulite and, 215–16
  digestive disorders and, 90
  to eat, 49–52, 71, 119, 124–25
  healing, 43–44
  thyroid function and, 63–66, 71
Fiber, 17–18, 21
  colon cleanse recipes and products,
    219–20
  constipation and, 217
  gallstones and, 135–36
Fibromyalgia, 92–94
  syndrome questionnaire, 92, 107–9
Field, Meira, 27
Fish, 52–53, 118, 122–23. *See also* Recipes
  iodine in, 72, 73
  mercury in, 76
Fish oil, 52–53, 136
Flaxseed oil, 68
Fluoride, 63, 75–76
Food allergies, 84, 217
Food cravings. *See* Sugar cravings
Frahm, David, 69
Frittatas, recipes, 158, 282–83
Fructose, 26–27
Fruits and vegetables. *See also specific fruits and*
    vegetables
  to avoid, 129, 130–31, 238
  to eat, 21, 37, 114, 119, 120–21, 125–26
  glycemic index and, 30
  reintroducing to diet, 235, 236–37

Gallbladder cleansing, 214, 228–32
  recipes and products, 231–32
Gallstones, 135–36, 229
Gastritis, 90
Gastrointestinal system, 89–91
Glucose (blood sugar), 29–34
  cravings and, 31–32
  glycemic index and, 29–31, 92
  sweeteners and, 24, 28
Glycemic index, 29–31, 92
Glycogen, 19, 20–21
Goals, setting, 99–100
Goitrogens, 63, 64–65, 74–75
Goldbecks' Guide to Good Food, 23
Grains, 20–21
  to avoid, 75, 129–30, 238, 275
  cooking tips, 240, 241
  fats in, 44–45
  nitrogen and, 126

  reintroducing to diet, 235, 237
  side dishes, recipes, 254–58
  thyroid and, 63, 113
Green tea, 36, 37, 118, 123–24

Halibut, recipes, 295–96
HDL cholesterol, 54
Health centers, resources, 301–3
Healthy carbs, x, 20–21, 235–72
  to avoid, 237–39
  basic preparation techniques, 239–41
  menu plan, 242–46
  recipes, 247–72
  reintroducing to diet, 236–37
Healthy fats, 114
Healthy rewards, 98–99
Heart disease, 12–13, 41, 44
  cholesterol and, 53–56
  factors contributing to, 56–57
Heavy metal detoxification, 73
Herbal supplements. *See* Supplements
Herxheimer reaction, 87–88
High-fat diets, 43, 51–52
Homocysteine, 54, 56–57
Honey, 24, 25
Hydrochloric acid, 85
Hydrogenation, 46, 47–49, 58
Hyperinsulinemia, 35
Hyperthyroidism, 61
Hypoglycemia, 97
Hypothyroidism, 59–62, 92, 94
  causes of, 63
  correcting problems, 69–70
  determining, 60–61
  fats and oils and, 63–66, 71
  symptoms, 59–60, 67, 69

Immune system
  candida and, 85–86
  chronic fatigue syndrome and, 92
  saturated fats and, 46
  sugar and, 22
Indigestion, 90
Inflammation, 54, 56
Inflammatory bowel disease (IBD), 90
Insulin, 28, 33–34, 223
Insulin resistance, 22, 34–35, 223
  fructose and, 27
  natural sweeteners and, 24
  quiz, 35, 39–40
Insulin sensitivity, 35–38

Introducing healthy carbs (phase III). *See* Healthy carbs
Iodine, 57, 63, 64–65, 72, 74, 77, 127
Irritable bowel syndrome (IBS), 90

Jenkins, David, 29
Joint problems, 114
Juicing (juices), 131–35
    menu plan, 132–33
    recipes, 133–35, 220, 226, 231–32, 234
    for thyroid health, 73–74

Kabara, Jon, 9
Kelp, 72, 73
Kendrick, Malcolm, 53
Kidney cleansing, 214, 233–34
    recipes and products, 234, 300
Koop, C. Everett, 15

Lauric acid, 9–10, 84–85
LCTs (long-chain triglycerides), 6–7, 15, 48–52, 65–67, 69
LDL cholesterol, 54
Lecithin, 228
Legumes, 118, 119, 120–21, 125–26
    cooking tips, 239–40
    fats and, 44–45
    insulin sensitivity and, 37
    starches in, 20–21, 30
Lemon, 230, 231. *See also* Recipes
Linoleic acid, 48–51
Lipid hypothesis, 12–13
Lipids, 44–45. *See also* Fats
Lipotropic formula, 232, 301
Liver cleansing, 76, 214, 222–28
    candida and, 86–87
    menu plan, 224–25
    recipes and products, 226–28, 300
Liver dysfunction, symptoms, 224
Lo Han Guo, 23–24
Long chain triglycerides (LCTs), 6–7, 15, 48–52, 65–67, 69
Low-carb diets, 21, 81–82, 89–90, 92
Low-carb natural sweeteners, 23–24
Low-carb vegetable juices, recipes, 133–35
Low-carb weight loss program. *See* 21-Day Weight Loss Diet
Low-fat diets, 41–42, 45, 51–52
Low stomach acid, 85
Low thyroid. *See* Hypothyroidism

L-tyrosine, 73
Lymphasizers, 76–77, 116, 216

Magnesium, 92–93
Malitol, 23
Maltose, 24
Mann, George, 53
Mannitol, 23
Maple syrup, 25, 27
Margarine, 43, 47–48, 64, 71, 129
Medium-chain triglycerides (MCTs), 6–9, 48–52, 55, 66, 71
Menopause, 5, 116
Menu plans
    1-Day Colon Cleanse, 218, 219
    1-Day Vegetable Juice Cleanse, 132–33
    7-Day Gallbladder Flush, 230
    7-Day Healthy Carbs, 242–46
    7-Day Kidney Flush, 233
    7-Day Liver Cleanse, 224–25
    7-Day Weight Maintenance, 276–80
    21-Day Weight Loss Diet, 136–51
Mercury, 63, 72, 73, 75–76
Milk and dairy, 118, 119
    to avoid, 128–29, 237, 274
    candida and, 84
    reintroducing to diet, 236
Milk thistle, 227
Minerals. *See* Supplements; *and specific minerals*
Molasses, 25–26
Monolaurin, 10
Monosaccharides, 18
Moussaka, 72
Murray, Michael, 86–87

National Cancer Institute (NCI), 62
National Heart Savers Association, 14
Natural sweeteners, 21, 23–26
Nettles tea, 234
Nicotine, 35–36
Nitrogen, 126
Norepinephrine, 31–32
NutraSweet, 28
Nuts, 73, 118, 119–20

Obesity, 41–44, 48–49, 58
Oils, 38, 44–45. *See also* Fats
    to avoid, 57–58, 274–75
    cellulite and, 215–16
    to eat, 49–52, 71, 119, 124–25

insulin sensitivity and, 37
oxidative stress and, 67, 69
thyroid function and, 63–66, 71
Olive oil, 71, 124, 125, 231
Omega-3 fatty acids, 36, 37, 46, 52–53
Omega-6 fatty acids, 52–53, 54
Organic foods, 50–51, 72, 126–27
Oxidative stress, 67, 69

Pancreas, 90
Peanut butter, 75
Peat, Ray, 48–51, 64, 67, 68, 69
Pesticides, 63, 126–27
Phase I. *See* 21-Day Weight Loss Diet
Phase II. *See* Cleansing
Phase III. *See* Healthy carbs
Phase IV. *See* Weight maintenance
Phytoestrogens, 64–65
Pizzorno, Joseph, 86–87
PMS, 31, 60, 94, 114
Polysaccharides, 18, 20–21
Polyunsaturated oils, 46, 47–49, 57–58
cholesterol and, 53
thyroid and, 63–66, 71
Potatoes, 20–21, 29, 33, 126, 130, 238
Poultry. *See* Chicken; Turkey
Price, Weston, 10
Probiotics, 82, 87, 220–21, 301
Progesterone, 67
Protein, 113, 118, 122–23
to avoid, 128, 274
blood sugar and, 37
CLA levels and, 50–51
heart disease and, 56
Psyllium fiber, 219–20

Quinoa, recipes, 254–55, 262–63
Quizzes
candida, 22, 87, 101–6
fibromyalgia syndrome, 92, 107–9
insulin resistance, 35, 39–40
thyroid, 59, 60, 78–80

Radishes, 73
Ravnskov, Uffe, 53
Rebounders, 116
Recipes
Aioli (Garlic Mayonnaise), 208–9
Almond Milk, 207
Apple-Pecan Turkey Salad, 249

Artichokes with Hollandaise Sauce, 181–82
Asian Citrus Dressing, 250
Asian Pesto, 209
Asian Scramble, 156
Avocado and Cream Cheese Frittata, 282–83
Baked Drumsticks with Spicy Eggplant, 201–2
Baked Lemon Chicken Thighs, 198
Basic Cheese Omelet, 157
Basic Frittata, 158
Basic Gazpacho, 177–78
Basic Scrambled Eggs, 154
Basic Vinaigrette, 172
Béchamel Sauce with Almond Milk, 268–69
Béchamel Sauce with Coconut Milk, 269
Béchamel Sauce with Dairy, 270
Beef Roll-Ups, 210–11
Beet Salad, 226, 232
Beet-Sauerkraut Salad, 170–71
Black Cherry Juice and Water, 220
Bouquet Garni, 210
Bread Machine Bread with Coconut Oil, 257
Brown Basmati Coconut Pilaf, 255–56
Butternut Squash, Sage, and Blue Cheese Gratin, 290
Caper and Egg Vinaigrette, 173
Caramelized Onion and Squash Gratin, 291
Carrot-Pineapple Slaw, 289
Carrot Salad with Lemon-Olive Oil Dressing, 226
Chef's Cheezy Eggs, 281
Chicken Breasts in Chunky Tomato-Vegetable Sauce, 202–3
Chicken Curry, 260–61
Chicken in Coconut Milk with Lime Leaves, 189–90
Chicken Salad, 171–72
Chicken Salad Stuffed Tomato, 164
Chicken with Citrus-Garlic-Ginger Sauce, 183–84
Chili, 184–85
Chipotle Lime Sour Cream Dip, 293
Citrus-Balsamic Vinaigrette, 251–52, 283
Classic Blender Hollandaise Sauce, 160, 182
Coconut Carrot Muffins, 258
Coconut Milk, Homemade, 206–7
Coconut Pineapple Sorbet, 272
Coconut Ranch Dressing, 252
Coconut Treats, 211–12
Cold Cucumber Avocado Soup, 134–35
Colon Cleanse Juice Cocktail, 220
Cornbread, 256–57
Cream of 4-Mushroom Soup, 286–87

Recipes *(continued)*
Creamy Vegetable Soup, 253–54
Creamy Vinaigrette, 249–50
Crispy Coconut Chicken Salad, 162–63
Curried Chicken Grape Salad, 284
Curried Chicken Salad, 171–72
Eggs Benedict Florentine, 160
Eggs Benedict with Turkey Ham, 159
Eggs Benedict Oscar, 160
Feather Light Coconut Macaroons, 271
Fiber Shake, 220
Fish in Fennel Sauce, 186–87
Gallbladder Cleansing Cocktail, 231
Garlic Mayonnaise (Aioli), 208–9
Garlic-Parmesan Halibut, 295–96
Garlic Vinaigrette, 173–74
Gazpacho Relish, 177–78
Golden Chicken, 188–89
Green Drink, 226
Grilled Lamb Salad, 166–67
Healthy Hamburgers, 185–86
Hollandaise Sauce, Classic Blender, 160, 182
Indian Coconut Vegetable Curry, 261–62
Jicama Pancakes, 247
Kidney Tonic, 234
Lamb and Eggplant Casserole, 192–93
Lemon-Chive Vinaigrette, 174
Lemon Curry Dressing, 171
Lemon Tarragon Fish, 196
Lemon Vinaigrette, 163–64
Low-Carb Coconut Smoothie, 153
Marinated Steak, 199
Minted Balsamic Dressing, 165
Morning Energy Cocktail, 133
Mustard Vinaigrette, 175
Napa Cabbage-Carrot Salad, 167–68
Nettles Tea, 234
Pico de Gallo, 204
Potassium-Rich Vegetable Broth, 227
Quinoa Millet Croquettes, 254–55
Quinoa-Stuffed Acorn Squash, 262–63
Roasted Squash with Poblano Pepper and
    Jack Cheese Quesadillas, 292–93
Salmon Steaks with Vegetables, 194–95
Sautéed Chicken Breasts with Pico de Gallo,
    203–4
Sautéed Chicken Breasts with Tomato Sauce,
    205–6
Simple Olive Oil Mayonnaise, 168
South-of-the-Border Scrambled Eggs,
    154–55
Southwestern Black Bean Soup, 285–86
Spicy Tomato on Ice, 134

Spinach Avocado Salad with Citrus-Balsamic
    Vinaigrette, 251–52
Steamed Eggs, 248
Steamed Vegetable Salad, 169–70
Stuffed Beef Rolls, 197–98
Stuffed Rainbow Trout Filets, 190–92
Super-Speedy Supper, 195
Tarragon Vinaigrette, 175–76
Tasty Greens Sauté, 180–81
Thai Chicken Soup with Coconut and
    Galanga, 178–79
Thai Coconut Salmon Over Wild and Brown
    Rice, 259
Thai Green Vegetable Curry, 294–95
Tomato Basil Soup, 288
Tomato-Herb Vinaigrette, 176
Tomato Sauce, 206
Turkey in Coconut Milk, 200–201
Turkey Roll-Ups, 210–11
Turkey Stew, 179–80
Unbelievable Baked Eggs, 162
Vegetable Quiche On-the-Go, 161
Veggie Scramble, 155
Virgin Coconut Oil Mayonnaise, 208
Wild Rice and Butternut Squash Pilaf,
    293–94
Yogurt Garlic Sauce, 264–65
Yogurt Sauce with Curry, 265
Yogurt Sauce with Feta Cheese, 266
Yogurt Sauce with Lemon, 264
Yogurt Sauce with Lime-Cilantro,
    266–67
Yogurt Sauce with Mint and Carrots, 267
Yogurt Sauce with Mint and Garlic, 268
Red meat, 113, 118, 122–23
    to avoid, 128, 274
    CLA and, 50–51
    heart disease and, 56
Refined sweeteners, 21–22, 26–27
Rescue Remedy, 117
Resources, 297–303
Rethinam, P., 11–12
Rice, 20–21, 29, 33
    cooking tips, 239, 241
    recipes, 259, 293–94
Rice cakes, 18–19, 29
Rosedale, Ron, 19, 33
Russell, Rex, 43

Safflower oil, 10–11
Salads and dressings, recipes, 162–76, 226,
    249–52, 283–84

Salmon, recipes, 194–95, 259
Salt, 63, 72, 127
Saturated fats, 38, 42–44, 57–58
    benefits of, 46–47
    cholesterol and, 53–56
Sauces, recipes, 264–70
Sea salt, 72, 127
Seeds, 44–45, 52, 119–20
Selenium, 73
Serotonin, 94–95
Silymarin, 227
Simple carbohydrates, 18–20, 22, 29, 37,
    41–43
Sleep, for weight loss, 116–17
Smoking, 35–36
Smoothies, 71, 153
Snack foods, 29, 130, 215, 238–39, 275
Sokolof, Phil, 14
Sorbitol, 23
Soups, recipes, 177–80, 253–54, 285–88
Soybeans, 14, 48–49, 52, 63, 64–65, 71
Soy oil, 47, 63, 64–65, 71, 74–75
Spices, 127, 210
Splenda, 28
Squash, recipes, 262–63, 290–94
Starches, 17–18, 20–21, 30
Stevia, 24, 75
Stress, 36, 38, 75, 94, 217
Sucralose, 28
Sugar alcohols, 23
Sugarcane, 26
Sugar cravings, 20, 31–32, 114–15
Sugars. *See* Sweeteners
Sugar substitutes, 27–29
Sunflower oil, 10–11
Supplements, 72–73, 121
    for gallbladder, 232
    for kidney, 233, 234, 300
    for liver, 228, 300
    resources, 300–301
Sweeteners, 17–19, 21–32
    artificial, 27–29, 35–36
    to avoid, 35, 239
    best, 118, 120, 128
    glycemic index and, 29–31
    natural, 21, 23–26
    refined, 21–22, 26–27
Sweet 'n' Low, 28
Sweet One, 28–29
Sweets, 35, 113, 130, 275
Symptoms
    candidiasis, 83
    gallbladder congestion, 228–29

hypothyroidism, 59–60, 67, 69
liver dysfunction, 224

Table syrup, 27
Taubes, Gary, 42–43
Textured vegetable protein, 74–75
Thampan, P. K., 11
Thermogenesis, 7, 49–50, 123
Thompson, Tommy G., 41
Thyroid, 59–80, 92. *See also* Hypothyroidism
    correcting problems, 69–70
    fats and oils and, 63–66, 71
    health quiz, 59, 60, 78–80
    homocysteine and, 56–57
    juicing for, 73–74
    lifestyle modifications, 74–77
    nourishing the, 70–74
    resources, 301
    supplements for, 72–73
Thyroid cancer, 62
Thyroid hormone replacement medications,
    69–70
Thyroid stimulating hormone (TSH), 61–62,
    67, 69
Tomatoes, 121, 125. *See also* Recipes
Toothpaste, 63, 76
Toxic oils, 46, 47–48
Trans-fatty acids, 47–48, 58
Trans-vaccenic acid, 51
Tropical diets, 3–8, 10–12, 46
    candida and, 85
    coconuts as staple, 3–6
    health secrets of, 8–10
Turkey, recipes, 159, 179–80, 200–201, 210–11,
    249

Vegetable dishes, recipes, 180–82, 289–95
Vegetable juice recipes, 133–35
Vegetable juices. *See* Juicing
Vegetables. *See* Fruits and vegetables
Vitamin A, 72–73, 136
Vitamin C, 22, 30, 117, 136
Vitamin D, 53
Vitamin E, 136
Vitamins. *See* Supplements; *and specific
    vitamins*

Walker, Shonagh, 216
Water, drinking, 87, 124, 136–37
Weight gain, gallbladder and, 228–29

Weight loss, 81–82, 113–17. *See also* 21-Day
    Weight Loss Diet
  coconut oil as secret to, 6–8
  constipation and, 217
  exercise and, 115–16
  gallstones and, 135–36
  green tea and, 36
  MCTs and, 6–9, 48–52
  natural sweeteners and, 24–26, 28
  sleep for, 116–17
  slimming fats, 49–52
Weight maintenance, x–xi, 273–96
  blood sugar and, 33
  carbohydrates and, 18–19

  foods to avoid, 274–76
  menu plan, 276–80
  recipes, 281–96
White bread, 19, 29, 75
White sugar, 26
Willett, Walter, 42–43
Williamson, Ehrlich, 28
Worst carbs, 18–20, 29

Xylitol, 23

Yeasts, 22, 82. *See also* Candida

About the Authors

CHERIE CALBOM, M.S., is known as a leading expert on nutrition, She earned a master of science degree in nutrition from Bastyr University, where she now sits on the Board of Regents. She frequently appears on QVC and speaks nationwide on the benefits of juicing and healthy living. She has written 14 books. Her best-selling book *Juicing for Life* has sold over 1.5 million copies. Cherie lives with her husband in Evergreen, Colorado.

JOHN CALBOM, M.A., is director of Trinity Retreat house, president of Trinity Wellness Institute, and a certified HeartMath provider. He is a behavioral medicine specialist, psychotherapist, and Eastern Orthodox priest. He was vice presisdent of St. Luke Medical Center and worked as a behavioral medicine therapist in complementary and preventative medicine.